Life with AIDS

Life with AIDS

Rose Weitz

Rutgers University Press
New Brunswick, New Jersey

Second paperback printing, 1992

Library of Congress Cataloging-in-Publication Data

Weitz, Rose, 1952–
     Life with AIDS / Rose Weitz.
          p.   cm.
     Includes bibliographical references and index.
     ISBN 0-8135-1629-3 (cloth)   ISBN 0-8135-1630-7 (pbk.)
          1. AIDS (Disease)—Psychological aspects.   2. AIDS (Disease)—
     Social aspects.   I. Title.
RC607.A26W45   1991
362.1'969792—dc20   90-36219
                                                                  CIP

British Cataloging-in-Publication information available

For Lilly Weitz, my mother,
and the memory of Bernard Weitz, my father

Contents

Preface and Acknowledgments

This book had its genesis one evening when I attended the annual meeting of our local chapter of the American Civil Liberties Union. The speaker that evening was attorney and professor Jane Aiken. Jane spoke of the discrimination and other troubles experienced by persons with AIDS and other stages of HIV disease and of her work protecting their civil rights.

As a medical sociologist, I had been following news of this illness for some time. Until that evening, however, I thought of it simply as a medical curiosity and not as something that had any unusual sociological or political ramifications. Jane's talk was riveting, and convinced me to learn more.

Shortly thereafter, Jane and I met for dinner, purely for social purposes (or at least so I thought). She told me that, contrary to my assumptions, almost no social scientists had yet begun researching HIV disease, and she urged me to do so. That remark was the start of this book. I am indebted to Jane for providing the impetus that began this project, assisting me whenever I had questions about the law and HIV, and letting me know at various crucial times that I was doing important work.

I would also like to thank the Arizona State Disease Control Research Commission and the College of Liberal Arts and Sciences of Arizona State University for their financial support of this project. In addition, the Department of Sociology of Arizona State University provided the day-to-day resources that made this work possible.

Portions of Chapter 4 appeared previously in "Uncertainty in the Lives of Persons with AIDS," *Journal of Health and Social Behavior* 30 (1989):270–281, and portions of Chapter 6 in "Living with the Stigma of AIDS," *Qualitative Sociology* 13 (1990):23–38 . Appendix 1 is a slightly revised version of "The Interview as Legacy: A Social Scientist Confronts AIDS," *Hastings Center Report* 17 (1987):21–23. I am grateful to the publishers for permission to reprint these materials.

I would also like to thank the Arizona AIDS Project, Phoenix Shanti Group, Tucson AIDS Project, Tucson Shanti Group, and the University Medical Center Infectious Disease Clinic for helping me to contact persons who have HIV disease. Without their assistance, this research would have been impossible.

My work on this book was eased by the several students who contributed their research assistance: Kathleen Abbott, Melissa Bolyard, Connie Brachtenbach, Rebecca Harrison, Shirley Philp, and Diane Wysocki. In addition, Barry Adam, Ed Kain, Nancy Shaw, Michelle St. Germain, and Deborah Sullivan gave me the benefit of their comments on several early draft chapters, Douglas Jardine and Pamela Wagner helped with editing the manuscript, and Bertram Jacobs graciously answered many questions about the microbiology of HIV.

I especially want to thank Peter Conrad and Martin Levine for their detailed comments on the draft manuscript; for their continual support and encouragement of this project, especially in its early stages; and for their friendship. Their help and support have meant more to me than they could ever know.

I am, as always, grateful for the love and good humor of my husband, Mark Pry, and the friendship of Miriam Axelrod, which sustained me through the completion of this project.

Finally, I would like to thank the persons with HIV disease and the doctors whom I interviewed for sharing their time and thoughts with me. I hope that this book justifies their trust.

Life with AIDS

CHAPTER 1

Introduction

He spoke quietly, with an air of resignation occasionally punctuated by expressions of bitterness. We sat at a dinette table, in an apartment he shared with his lover. By Arizona standards, the apartment and neighborhood were old, developed in the 1960s. The dining area was just a corner of the living room, the kitchen an alcove off the dining area. The room's only window looked out onto the street. The apartment was furnished with an uncoordinated assortment of chairs and tables that had been donated by friends and relatives. The nondescript interior suggested temporary quarters established under straitened circumstances; the single object in the living room that conveyed any sense of individuality was an unfinished quilt lying on a rack near the window.

"My life is like an hourglass," Jeremy said.[1] "And I think life always is an hourglass, but I think now you really recognize it. It's going right in front of you. You are watching the grains go through, and as grains go through, they fall. And there is a lot of falling, it's a lot of things that really throw you. Real depressing, kind of falling feeling."

Jeremy had learned he had AIDS seven months before. Although the illness frequently makes its sufferers appear much older than they actually are, Jeremy, who was twenty-six, still looked like a teenager. He was slim, with delicate features, and he walked

1

and gestured gracefully. He enjoyed talking, though much of his story was painful, both to tell and to hear.

I had first spoken with Jeremy six months ago, one month after he had been diagnosed as having AIDS. Much had changed since then. During the first interview, he was warm, effervescent, and witty. Although he had lost fifteen pounds from his already-slim frame, he seemed otherwise healthy and lively. He spoke energetically and rapidly, rarely stopping to think about how to answer a question, and frequently used his hands for emphasis. He occasionally expressed anger at how his co-workers and relations had reacted to his illness, but he also found much humor in his situation. And although he already had been hospitalized once, his situation did not seem very threatening to him. At one point, his doctor had expressed surprise that Jeremy was taking his diagnosis so well. His response, as he told me, was a straightforward one. "What am I supposed to do?" he recalled telling his doctor. "I mean, I have AIDS. I have to continue on with the rest of my life. I'm going to have to make changes, but I'm not going to be devastated by this."

By the time I revisited him for our second interview six months later, Jeremy had acknowledged the gravity of his situation. His health had deteriorated significantly. At the time of the first interview, he had believed that he would live for at least another year; now, however, he believed his chances of surviving the remaining six months of that year were only about 60 percent. As a result, he was devoting more of his time and attention to unrealized goals. The quilt was a project that he and his lover had been talking about sewing together for some time. Recently Jeremy had decided that they either had to start the quilt or risk not finishing it.

Jeremy's social situation also had deteriorated. His relationship with his lover was strained, for the lover refused to acknowledge that Jeremy was seriously ill or even to talk about Jeremy's illness. One friend had died of AIDS. Another was hospitalized. Several others had broken off contact with Jeremy as his illness had progressed. His co-workers had made their fears and hostility so obvious that he could no longer tolerate the stress of working. Once he quit his job, his former employer cancelled his health insurance immediately, without giving him the time required by law to find alternative coverage. He subsequently had to apply for public assistance to pay his living expenses and for publicly funded medical insurance to pay his bills. Both forms of assistance had been slow in coming, and neither was quite sufficient, so each month he found himself further in debt. He was losing control of his life to AIDS, and he knew it.

Between 1986 and 1989, I conducted semi-structured interviews with thirty-seven men and women living in Arizona who had HIV disease. The term *HIV disease* refers to all stages of illness caused by infection with human immunodeficiency virus (HIV). One of these stages is Acquired Immune Deficiency Syndrome (AIDS). Some of the people I interviewed had AIDS; some had AIDS-Related Complex (ARC), a diagnostic category that includes persons who do not fit the narrow definition of AIDS but may have other life-threatening illnesses caused by HIV; and some simply were infected with HIV. Of the last group, some had experienced ill health as a result of HIV and some had not. I reinterviewed thirteen of these people four to six months after their initial interviews. (For further methodological details, see Appendix 2.)

The stories these persons told me all demonstrated how both the physical realities of HIV disease and the social reactions to it can tear apart people's lives. Yet few of the people I spoke with were passive victims of HIV. Instead, they strove to find reasons for what was happening to them, to fight for their physical and emotional health, and to make their lives worth living despite their illness. My purpose in this book is to describe how the lives of persons with HIV disease change as a result of their illness and how they cope with these changes. I present a holistic picture of the experiences of persons with HIV disease, using their own words wherever appropriate and focusing on the issues that they consider important. The central chapters of this book reflect the central concerns of these persons, describing how they are affected by and respond to their illness, from the time they realize that they are at risk to the time death approaches. Because the effects of HIV disease spread far beyond those who have the illness, I also include a chapter on how doctors are affected by and cope with the unique pressures of treating HIV disease.

This book differs from previous writings about HIV disease in that it brings the concerns of those who live with HIV to the forefront. Previous research on doctors has focused almost solely on explaining why so few doctors will treat persons infected with HIV[2]; almost none has looked at what happens to those who do. Similarly, despite all that has been written about this illness, we still know surprisingly little about how HIV disease has affected the social rather than simply the physical lives of infected persons. This social aspect has been underreported in the mass media, in medical journals, and, surprisingly, even in social scientific journals.

As the next chapter discusses, the mass media initially ignored HIV disease, assuming that it threatened only gay men. Coverage expanded significantly once it became clear that heterosexuals also could become infected. However, although that wider coverage has helped educate the public about the biology of HIV disease, it has not given a clear picture of the lives of infected persons. The mass media, for the most part, have elected to present anecdotal, and relatively superficial, coverage, rather than in-depth analysis. They also have focused on news-breaking events rather than ongoing situations—the discovery of a new drug to treat HIV disease, for example, but not the everyday problems faced by persons who have this illness. Moreover, because the media are commercial enterprises, when they have investigated the lives of persons with HIV disease, they typically have highlighted those aspects that will attract or titillate readers—esoteric sexual practices, bizarre clinical manifestations, and the grim tragedies of deaths among babies and others whom the public considers "innocent" victims of this illness. Such coverage cannot provide us with a clear picture of what daily life is like for most persons with HIV disease.

Nor have scholarly researchers shown us what life is like for persons with HIV disease. Medical researchers have focused on how this illness affects individuals' vital organs and immune systems rather than on how it affects their everyday lives. The federal government, meanwhile, has shown little interest in funding social science research on HIV disease. Most social scientists who, despite the poor chances for funding, are researching this illness have limited themselves to studying the conditions under which people change their sexual or drug-using behavior. Consequently, there is now a substantial literature on how gay men have changed their sexual activities in response to the threat of HIV and a growing literature on how drug users are attempting to reduce their risks of becoming infected.

Within this narrow framework, most social scientists have adopted an even narrower focus, investigating individual predictors of sexual behavior or needle-sharing but not looking at these behaviors in a broader cultural context. Many researchers, for example, have investigated how often gay men engage in various forms of sexual activity or how often drug users share needles. Few, however, have asked what those activities mean to the participants, what benefits they receive from these activities beyond physical gratification, or what role these behaviors play in their subcultures. Moreover, because these studies tend to look solely at individual behavior without investigating its social context, they do not recognize the legal, social, economic, and cultural barriers that might prevent individuals from adopting safer behaviors. For example, drug users may risk arrest if they carry their own needles instead of borrowing or renting them, and women may risk beatings if they ask their lovers to use condoms.

Although these medical social scientific studies have helped in developing public health strategies for dealing with HIV disease, unintentionally they dehumanize persons with this illness. They do so in a variety of ways: by reducing them to unthinking and unfeeling bloodstreams, sexual organs, or neurological systems; by focusing almost solely on the non-normative aspects of their lives; and by emphasizing how individuals place themselves and others at risk. Consequently, such research implicitly, although unintentionally, suggests that persons with HIV disease not only deserve their illness but also are a dangerous and inherently alien "other" whose actions should be watched and if necessary controlled for the sake of the majority.

Until recently, such research, which took the perspective of the medical world and at times painted the ill as deviant, was the norm for most sociologists who studied illness. Those few who did take the perspective of the ill typically focused on ill persons as patients and on their relationships with health care providers.[3] Yet whether the illness is acute or chronic, major or minor, most of the experience of illness occurs in the everyday world where one lives, works, and loves, rather than in doctors' offices or hospitals.[4]

The last decade has seen a growing interest among sociologists in how people live with illness and a shift away from a more medicalized interest in the social causes and distribution of disease.[5] To social scientists, "disease" refers to specific, physical changes in the body and "illness" to how those changes (whether real or perceived) are understood and experienced by ill persons and others. Ill persons, then, may be said to *have* a disease but to *live* with an illness. This book adds to the developing literature on illness experience by looking at the everyday world of persons with HIV disease, highlighting both the similarities and the differences between living with HIV disease and living with other illnesses.

I chose to conduct this research in Arizona for practical reasons. Nevertheless, there are good intellectual reasons for this choice as well. As of November 1989, Arizona ranked twenty-second out of the fifty states in the number of reported AIDS cases.[6] (No reports are kept of the total number of persons with HIV disease.) Arizona's rate of 8.4 cases per 100,000 (compared, for example, to New York's rate of 36.4 and Idaho's rate of 2.1) also places it in the middle of the national rankings. Arizona is thus not one of the states (such as New York, California, and Florida) where HIV initially took root, but it will be one of the many states that will be hard hit by HIV in the near future. To date, however, most research on HIV disease has taken place in the states with the initial nuclei of cases. Research conducted in Arizona, therefore, can help us understand what life is like for persons with HIV disease and their doctors in areas where HIV is just beginning to have an impact, where legislatures and electorates are conservative, where social services are underdeveloped, and where the gay community is politically weak. Thus, studying HIV disease in Arizona provides us with clues regarding what the future will be like, as the disease spreads inward from the current centers of infection on the two coasts to the American heartland.

These Arizona data must be put into context, however. The distribution of HIV disease in the United States follows two distinct patterns. On the East Coast, intravenous drug users and their sexual partners comprise a substantial minority of persons with HIV disease (and a majority within certain areas such as New York City). On the West Coast, although the proportion of cases attributable to drug use is growing, the overwhelming majority of persons with HIV disease still are gay men. Arizona, not surprisingly, conforms to the West Coast pattern: 73 percent of Arizona men with AIDS, compared to 63 percent of U.S. men with AIDS, are homosexual or bisexual men who have not used drugs, and only 35 percent of Arizona women with AIDS, compared to 53 percent of U.S. women with AIDS, are drug users.[7] Because drug use is not an important means of transmitting HIV disease in Arizona, a higher percentage of persons with HIV disease in Arizona than in the U.S. as a whole are white (86 percent in Arizona versus 59 percent elsewhere) and slightly fewer are women (6 percent versus 10 percent). Thus, the findings presented in this book will be most easily extrapolated to other western and midwestern states, with moderate incidences of HIV disease, that follow the West Coast infection pattern.

Overview of Book

To understand individuals' experiences of illness, we first have to understand the social context in which those experiences occur.

Thus, in the next chapter, I review the history and biology of HIV disease, analyze why HIV disease has produced the social reactions it has, and discuss some of the consequences of those reactions. Chapter 3 puts HIV disease in broader context, by exploring the moral status of illness and looking at why some illnesses, including HIV disease, have become especially stigmatized. The next four chapters look specifically at the lives of persons with HIV disease, drawing on the interviews I conducted. Chapter 4 explores how, before diagnosis, individuals assess their risks of infection and the meaning of any symptoms they exhibit, how they obtain a diagnosis, and how they develop their initial ideas about the consequences of HIV disease for their futures. Chapter 5 describes the impact of HIV disease on the body, and how the lives and self-concepts of persons with HIV disease change as their bodies change. Chapter 6 describes how HIV disease affects social relationships. Chapter 7 explores how persons with HIV disease come to terms with their ailing bodies, changed social relationships, and impending deaths. Chapter 8 takes a different tack, looking at how these and other problems affect doctors who treat persons with HIV disease and how these doctors cope with their situations. This chapter draws on semi-structured interviews I conducted with twenty-six Arizona doctors (both primary practitioners and specialists) who had treated anywhere from three to several hundred persons with HIV disease. The concluding chapter theorizes about how changes in the social construction, demographic distribution, and treatment of HIV disease are changing the lives of persons who have this illness. Finally, Appendix 1 describes the ethical, legal, and personal problems I faced in interviewing ill or dying persons who have an infectious and stigmatized illness, and Appendix 2 describes my methodology.

A Note on Terminology

There is no standard way to refer to either those who have HIV disease or their illness. When I began doing this research, both popular and scientific discourse on the subject focused largely on persons with AIDS (commonly called PWAs) rather than on the range of persons infected with HIV—from those who are asymptomatic to those who are dying of full-blown AIDS. No term existed for all those infected with HIV, and HIV itself was commonly called "the AIDS virus" rather than its technical name. Although many people (particularly nonscientists) still use the term *AIDS* to refer to the full spectrum of health problems caused by HIV, clinicians and researchers increasingly are adopting the terms *HIV disease* or *HIV infection*. In this book, therefore, I have chosen to use the term *HIV disease*. I have retained the terms *AIDS* and *ARC* in quotations and citations to be true to my sources and have used the term *AIDS* in the title because it is still the most widely recognized; the reader will therefore find several places where persons who are asymptomatic but infected with HIV refer to themselves as having AIDS. Similarly, although it is awkward, I use the term *persons with HIV disease* to refer to all persons infected with HIV. Where appropriate, I further describe individuals as asymptomatic, having chronic HIV infection (that is, relatively minor health problems caused by HIV), or having AIDS (that is, life-threatening health problems caused by HIV that meet the government's definition of full-blown AIDS).

In writing this book, I also had to decide how to refer to the individuals I interviewed. To protect those I spoke with, as well as their families, friends, lovers, and employers, I have used pseudonyms to refer to both persons with HIV disease and their doctors. To reinforce to the reader that these are pseudonyms, I have used only first names. Having decided to use only first names for persons with HIV disease, I realized that, for the sake of consistency, I should also use only first names for the doctors. I hope that no doctors are offended by this informality.

CHAPTER 2

The Social Construction of HIV Disease

HIV disease is biologically devastating, producing progressive physical and sometimes mental disability and the likelihood of an early death. Yet these stark facts alone cannot explain the government's apparent indifference toward, or the public's almost medieval dread of and accusations of blame against, persons with HIV disease. To understand the lives of persons who have this illness, therefore, we need to understand both the biology of this disease and its social construction as an illness, that is, the meanings society has given to it.

The Emergence of HIV and AIDS

The social construction of HIV disease and the ensuing responses to those who have it set it apart from all other modern illnesses. This social construction in large part reflects the unique history and biology of HIV disease.

Anecdotal reports of this illness first surfaced in 1979 among doctors working in New York, San Francisco, and Los Angeles. These doctors had noticed that Kaposi's sarcoma, a rare form of cancer that normally affects elderly heterosexual Italian and Jewish men, had begun appearing in young gay men. Moreover, whereas

10

Kaposi's sarcoma was usually a mild, chronic condition, these new gay patients became terribly disfigured by purple lesions and then rapidly died.

Over the next two years, another curious disease began attacking and killing gay men. This time the disease was *pneumocystis carinii* pneumonia (PCP), a rare form of pneumonia that generally affects only persons whose immune systems have been weakened by chemotherapy, certain serious illnesses, or drugs taken after organ transplants to suppress the immune system so it will not attack the "foreign" organ. In such circumstances, people cannot fight infections. They subsequently fall ill because various microorganisms that usually live benignly in the body take advantage of this opportunity to multiply. The resulting illnesses are known as opportunistic infections. On 5 June 1981, the Centers for Disease Control (CDC), which tracks the spread of disease in the United States, published the first official notice of the PCP outbreak.[1]

One month after the article on the PCP cases appeared, the CDC published a second article describing an outbreak of Kaposi's sarcoma among gay men, several of whom also had PCP.[2] CDC researchers subsequently spoke with doctors around the country to ascertain whether this was a new outbreak of Kaposi's sarcoma or whether cases like these had been appearing for years without anyone noticing the pattern. Their conversations convinced them that some new factor was at work. Further investigation confirmed that the rate of PCP also had increased suddenly. By definition, then, whatever disease had caused the outbreak of PCP and Kaposi's sarcoma was an epidemic—that is, a significant increase in, or first appearance of, cases of a disease. Because the orginal cases were all gay men, researchers unofficially began calling this new disease Gay Related Immune Disorder, or GRID. Thus researchers started the process of linking this new disease with homosexuality in people's thoughts.

At this point, no one knew what had caused this strange outbreak of opportunistic infections. Clearly, however, something had destroyed the immune systems of these men. The purpose of the immune system is to recognize and destroy any harmful substances that enter our bodies. The immune systems of persons with GRID had lost the ability to do so, leaving them susceptible to infection by virtually any microorganism in their environment. As a result, the men died quick and ugly deaths, their bodies overwhelmed by infections and their strength drained by coughing, nausea, diarrhea, fevers, and the like.

To understand what had caused this devastating illness, researchers sought to determine what persons with GRID had in common and how they differed from healthy gay men. The researchers discovered that the ill men had far higher numbers of sexual partners, especially anonymous sexual partners, and higher rates of venereal disease. The ill men also were more likely to use amyl nitrates ("poppers"), "fisting," and "rimming" (inserting or receiving fist or tongue into the anus) in their sexual encounters. Journalists' accounts of this early research contributed to the social construction of GRID as not only a "gay disease" but a disease of gay men whose lifestyles seemed particularly alien and depraved.

At this point, most scientists were convinced that the epidemic was caused by some new infectious agent. This theory gained credence when researchers discovered that several of the earliest cases had had sex with each other. These researchers hypothesized that a "fast-lane" sex life characterized the early cases because only those with many sexual partners would have come in contact with whatever rare germ or virus was causing the epidemic. A minority of scientists, however, concluded that these men had become ill because their constant exposure to semen, drugs, and sexually transmitted diseases had damaged their immune systems. Although this "overload" theory never won wide acceptance among scientists, publicity about the theory reinforced the popular notion that gay men were falling ill not because of a virus but because they chose to engage in unsafe behaviors. Thus, from an early point, the social construction of GRID emphasized that its sufferers had caused their own ill health. This view still underlies the responses of many members of the public to persons with HIV disease, as well as the way some persons with HIV disease view themselves.

Once researchers and clinicians realized that this illness did not affect only gay men, the overload theory became implausible. By 1982, doctors had identified cases of GRID in Haitian and African men who denied ever engaging in gay sex, as well as in heterosexual women, hemophiliacs, and persons who used illicit intravenous drugs. That these particular groups were falling ill indicated that the illness was transmitted through blood and semen and could infect anyone exposed to the virus, regardless of sexual orientation or lifestyle. Nevertheless, the assumption of a connection between homosexuality and GRID was so strong that when doctors first reported cases in children of drug users and in persons who had received blood transfusions, many influential doctors and members of the blood-banking industry refused to believe that these persons had GRID.[3] Only as the number of cases mounted inexorably did the medical establishment accept that this was indeed the case. Nevertheless, GRID still seemed to most Americans to be a disease of the "other." The only change was that now that "other" included drug users and black foreigners as well as a few unfortunate "innocent" victims.

Reflecting scientists' developing understanding of the epidemic, in September 1982 the CDC officially coined the term *Acquired Immune Deficiency Syndrome,* or AIDS, and established a clinical definition for the disease. Later, the CDC added a second diagnostic category of AIDS-Related Complex, or ARC, to include the many persons who had developed serious health problems as a result of the same underlying immune disorder but who had not met the CDC's definition of AIDS.

To trace the spread of AIDS, the CDC began requiring that U.S. doctors report all new cases to them. The number of reported AIDS cases (which probably represents less than two thirds of actual cases) passed 100,000 in July 1989, by which time the World Health Organization had received official reports of AIDS cases from 149 countries.[4]

In addition to reporting demographic information, doctors were required to assign each case to a "risk group," indicating the way the person was most likely to have become infected. The CDC's definitions of the various risk groups unintentionally reinforced the social construction of AIDS as primarily a gay disease and secondarily a disease of other deviants.[5] As originally defined by the CDC, gay men who also used intravenous drugs were to be reported simply as gay. Haitians, most of whom had contracted AIDS through heterosexual intercourse, were to be reported as Haitians rather than as heterosexuals. Even more than the category of "gay men," the Haitian risk group (later dropped by the CDC because of political pressure) referred not to what one did, had done, or might do, but simply to what one *was*. Both the original and the current CDC definitions still assign individuals to the heterosexual risk group only if they have no other risks and can identify a specific heterosexual lover with AIDS. For example, a woman who uses intravenous drugs and whose lover also uses intravenous drugs is reported simply as a drug user, and a woman who does not know how she became infected but has had many heterosexual lovers is categorized as having an unknown mode of transmission.[6] In all these ways, then, the definitions of the risk groups caused the CDC to overestimate the risk that gay male sexual activity would lead to AIDS and underestimate the risk that other behaviors, especially heterosexual behavior, would do so. Consequently, these definitions reinforced the social construction of AIDS as a gay disease.

The connection between deviance and AIDS was also reinforced in the public's mind by the CDC's terminology of "risk groups" rather than "risk behaviors."[7] This phrasing gave the impression that AIDS somehow sought out persons who belonged to certain communities, rather than striking persons who engaged in particular behaviors.[8] Those who did not belong to such groups, therefore, could easily conceptualize AIDS as an illness that only affected persons inherently different from themselves and from the majority of Americans. In addition, the emphasis on risk groups led Americans to believe that all members of these groups, regardless of their behaviors, were equally at risk and equally a threat to others. For example, many believe that lesbians are at high risk, even though doctors have only identified a handful of lesbians with

AIDS. Moreover, these few women probably contracted AIDS through intercourse with men (which most lesbians have had at some point in their lives) or drug use, rather than through lesbian activity; in general, sexually transmitted diseases are extremely rare among lesbians because lesbian activity is an ineffective transmitter of infections.[9]

Scientists' understanding of AIDS grew enormously following the isolation in May 1983 of Human Immunodeficiency Virus (HIV), the virus that causes AIDS. Two years later, researchers announced the development of a test to identify persons infected with the virus.

The existence of a test for exposure to HIV greatly facilitated research on its spread. Although many Americans have continued to regard HIV disease as a mysteriously threatening illness, researchers quickly learned that HIV is only spread through sexual intercourse; through sharing unclean intravenous needles; through some unclear mechanism from mother to fetus and, possibly, through breast milk from mother to infant; and through transfusions or accidental injections with blood or blood products. This last mode of transmission has become uncommon in the developed world since mid-1985, when blood banks began to test blood routinely for HIV.[10] Studies demonstrate conclusively that HIV is not spread through insects, spitting, sneezing, hugging, nonsexual touching, or even sharing eating utensils. Of the hundreds of friends and family members who have lived in households with persons who have HIV disease— sharing toothbrushes, beds, dishes, and the like—none has become infected except through sexual intercourse. Even regular sexual partners of persons with HIV disease often remain uninfected if they use condoms lubricated with spermicide.

As of November 1989, the majority (61 percent) of adult AIDS cases reported to the CDC have been traced to gay male activity. Twenty-one percent have occurred in intravenous drug users, 7 percent in persons who engage in both male homosexual activity and intravenous drug use, 3 percent in persons who have received contaminated transfusions with blood or blood products, and

5 percent in persons who have had heterosexual intercourse with persons who have HIV disease.[11] Eighty-one percent of children with AIDS were born to women with HIV disease and 16 percent received transfusions before the blood test for HIV became routine.

The World Health Organization now estimates that the rate of infection with HIV is about one hundred times greater than the rate of AIDS and that at least 21 million adults will be infected with HIV by the year 2000.[12] Current data suggest that most persons develop AIDS about ten years after they are infected with HIV.[13] No one yet knows whether all infected persons will develop AIDS, however. Nor does anyone know the maximum number of years it can take before an infected individual will develop AIDS, nor why some persons develop AIDS sooner than others, although some clear patterns have emerged—children, for example, generally develop AIDS much sooner after infection than do adults.

The realization that millions of seemingly healthy persons can transmit HIV has contributed greatly to the public's fear of HIV disease and eagerness to identify and distance themselves from those who are infected. In addition, the lack of certainty about how soon individuals will progress from infection with HIV to AIDS and from AIDS to death continues to exacerbate both the public's belief that AIDS is an especially mysterious and frightening illness and the psychological distress experienced by persons with HIV disease.

Throughout the 1980s, the prevailing consensus among researchers was that most and perhaps all infected persons would eventually die from either AIDS or some other illness caused by HIV. Because HIV was assumed to lead rapidly and ineluctably to AIDS, HIV and AIDS seemed almost synonymous, and were assumed to be synonymous by many members of the public and some persons with HIV disease. Entering the 1990s, new therapies have significantly improved the prognosis for persons with HIV disease. Some observers, especially clinicians and activists, now argue that HIV disease should be considered a chronic, manageable illness, rather than a fatal one. Others, especially those researchers who do not engage in direct patient care and are less emotionally involved, suspect that the life span of persons with HIV disease will continue to lengthen, but that HIV infection will remain a fatal illness for the foreseeable future.

This improved prognosis for persons with HIV disease has caused a parallel shift in the conceptualization of the disease itself. Clinicians, activists, and researchers agree that medicine's focus in the early years of epidemic on full-blown AIDS hindered our understanding of the disease as a whole. Authorities now agree that we need a new diagnostic model that will reflect the natural history of all the stages of HIV disease—from asymptomatic infection to the development of chronic, nonfatal health problems to life-threatening illnesses, including AIDS. Such a model would emphasize the millions of persons living with HIV disease rather than the much smaller number dying from AIDS.[14] Whether the public will accept this new conceptualization of HIV disease, and what impact this will have on its responses to persons with HIV disease, remain to be seen.

In sum, although many questions remain to be answered, scientists increasingly find HIV disease simply one more viral disease—a serious health problem, but comprehensible, manageable at least in the early stages, and no more a punishment from God than any other illness. Yet the social construction of HIV disease as a frightening, incomprehensible, and uncontrollable illness of deserving "others" remains. To understand why this social construction of HIV disease continues, we need to look not only at the unique history and biology of HIV, but also at how that history and biology have been presented to the public.

The Media and HIV Disease

The public derives most of its information about HIV disease from the mass media. Because the media initially considered HIV disease a "gay" disease, they provided little coverage of the topic during the first years of the epidemic.[15] The *New York Times,* for example, did not print a single story about AIDS during all of 1981 and printed only six stories in 1982, by which time more than two hundred Americans had died. In contrast, it printed 32 articles on toxic shock syndrome, 111 articles about cyanide-laced Tylenol capsules, and 86 articles about legionnaire's disease during the year in which each of those far less deadly problems first appeared.[16] The few reports of AIDS published in 1981 and 1982 typically described it as a gay disease. The first article on HIV disease to appear in a national magazine, for example, was entitled "The Gay Plague," and until 1983 both the *New York Times Index* and the *Readers' Guide to Periodical Literature* indexed articles on HIV disease only under the heading "homosexuality."[17] Thus, from the start, heterosexuals were taught to associate HIV disease with homosexuality.

The media's consistent focus on the more esoteric aspects of the lifestyles of persons with HIV disease further highlighted the differences between those groups considered at risk (especially gay men) and what the articles referred to as "the general population."[18] Sensationalist accounts of gay sexual activity and of addicts desperate for drugs enabled the public to distance themselves emotionally from those who had HIV disease and to see HIV as a threat primarily to persons inherently different from themselves.

In May 1983, Dr. Anthony Fauci, director of the National Institute of Allergy and Infectious Disease, published an editorial in the prestigious *Journal of the American Medical Association* in which he suggested that HIV theoretically might be transmitted through casual contact.[19] The editorial received substantial publicity, and news coverage of HIV disease increased significantly in the following weeks. However, reporters paid little attention to Fauci's subsequent statement that he had not meant that transmission through casual contact was likely.[20] Six months after the editorial, news coverage had dropped almost to its initial low level. This episode and its treatment in the media did not cause the public to stop thinking of HIV disease as a gay disease. Instead, the public now thought of HIV disease as a gay disease that threatened "normal people."

The social construction of HIV disease as a gay disease that now threatened others was reinforced by the media's frequent division of persons with HIV disease into the "innocent," the "suspect," and the "guilty."[21] Media accounts described children with HIV disease as "innocent victims" of a great tragedy who needed and deserved our compassion, while describing gay men and drug users with HIV disease in ways that encouraged a sense of distance or even horror rather than sympathy. Reports of Haitians with HIV disease (who already suffered stigma because of their poverty, race, and immigrant status) typically described them as suspect, by raising questions about whether they had lied to the government about their homosexual activity or drug use.

The social construction of HIV disease as an especially threatening illness was heightened by the media's reluctance to describe frankly the biological realities of the disease.[22] Until well into 1985, stories about the illness avoided words like *penis, intercourse,* and *semen* and instead euphemistically talked about "intimate sexual contact" and "exchange of bodily fluids." Many who read these stories became worried unnecessarily about contracting HIV disease through saliva, tears, or sweat spread by hugging, eating, or shaking hands.

The media also contributed to the fear of HIV disease through its questionable use of "experts."[23] Journalists are neither trained nor expected by their superiors to evaluate conflicting scientific claims. Rather, their job is to solicit and publish the views of various "authorities," without identifying one authority as more reliable than another. As a result, the media, in their attempt to present all sides of the story, have given substantial coverage to some highly questionable scientific theories.

Most importantly, and realizing that such sensationalist stories sell, the media have highlighted the few researchers who believe that HIV can be easily transmitted and will spread rapidly. For example, journalists eagerly reported the conclusions of well-known sex researchers William Masters, Virginia Johnson, and Robert Kolodny, who argue in a recent book that "the AIDS virus is now running rampant in the heterosexual community" and that HIV can be spread through a variety of means that CDC and the over-whelming majority of scientists consider unlikely or impossible—sports, blood transfusions, lesbian activity, insect bites, toilet seats, food prepared by an infected cook, and the like.[24] The media glossed over the authors' acknowledgment that these risks are small, unquantifiable, or even "farfetched" and that they have no confirming evidence.[25] Moreover, the media rarely mentioned that other scientists have considerable opposing evidence. In fulfilling their mandate as they see it and in presenting all views impartially, therefore, the media have misrepresented what science knows about HIV disease and have encouraged the public's fears.

That fear remains substantial. According to data collected in November 1988 through a national random sample, 30 percent of U.S. adults still considered it somewhat or very likely that a person could contract AIDS from "sharing plates, forks, or glasses with someone who has the AIDS virus."[26] Almost as many (25 percent) believed it likely that one could contract AIDS through insect bites or through "eating in a restaurant where the cook has the AIDS virus." Finally, 18 percent and 12 percent respectively believed it somewhat or very likely that AIDS can be transmitted by "using public toilets" or "working near someone with the AIDS virus." Even some persons with HIV disease share these ideas, and conse-quently live in fear of infecting those close to them.

Homophobia and the Response to HIV Disease

The social construction of HIV disease as a gay disease foisted on an unsuspecting public fed upon preexisting views of gay people as alien and inferior. At the time this illness first was identified, and in the years since then, homosexuality was and has remained a stig-matized activity. From 1973 to 1988, at least 70 percent of Ameri-cans in national surveys have agreed that homosexual activity is "always wrong."[27] In a national Gallup poll conducted in 1982, when news of AIDS was first appearing, 39 percent stated that homosexual relations between consenting adults should not be legal and 28 percent thought "homosexuals should . . . not have equal rights in terms of job opportunities."[28] This percentage rose to 59 percent when individuals were questioned about whether homosexuals should have equal rights in such sensitive occupations as elementary school teacher. Thus, many people were predisposed to stigmatize persons with HIV disease either as gays or as having a "gay disease."

These feelings have been exacerbated by right-wing leaders who have used the epidemic of HIV disease to promote their political agenda. HIV disease has become the focus for a symbolic crusade, an organized political campaign designed to enforce, or at least symbolically reaffirm, a particular group's values.[29] Such crusades develop when a group whose social values once dominated their society feel that they have lost that dominance. In his classic statement of this concept, for example, Joseph Gusfield argues that the temperance movement in the United States was started because native-born Americans of northern and western European descent wanted to reassert their political dominance and moral supremacy over the new immigrants from southern and eastern Europe, who brought with them very different attitudes toward the use of alcohol. These attitudes provided a convenient focus for a crusade whose true purpose was to reassert social dominance.

Similarly, the right wing's position on HIV disease essentially argues for reaffirming right-wing beliefs in marriage, heterosexuality, and a literal Christian tradition—beliefs that they feel have been abandoned or at least threatened by feminism and liberalism. Their arguments typically begin by asserting that the epidemic of HIV disease was caused by homosexuals. For example, archconservative columnist James K. Fitzpatrick writes:

> One thing is certain: You do not get AIDS the way people got polio. Near to 75 percent of those who get the disease are homosexuals. And the record is clear, the other cases are indirectly related to homosexuals. The drug users used a needle

once used by a homosexual. Others receive a blood transfusion from a homosexual, or from someone who received a transfusion from a homosexual. The children who become victims are children of homosexuals or bisexuals or drug users who contracted the disease from a homosexual. The disease is being spread by homosexuals to each other, and, increasingly, to the rest of society.[30]

Conservatives further assert that HIV disease is either "nature's revenge" or divine retribution for non-normative practices.[31] For example, Gene Antonio devotes much of his book, *The AIDS Cover-Up?*, to arguing that homosexuality is inherently unhealthy and leads inexorably to parasitical infections, hepatitis, syphilis, gastrointestinal disorders, and other health problems.[32] Meanwhile, others, such as the American Council of Christian Churches, have declared that AIDS is God's judgment against homosexuals.[33]

The most extreme members of the far right have claimed that gay men not only introduced HIV into the western world but did so as a deliberate form of "blood terrorism."[34] For example, Enrique Rueda and Michael Schwartz contend that gay leaders intentionally allowed HIV to spread because they "have not looked upon AIDS primarily as a health catastrophe, but as an opportunity to push forward their political agenda. . . . AIDS has become for the homosexual movement an ideological source of strength; a shared suffering that creates a sense of solidarity, a special identity, and a justification for claiming the status of victim and for demanding the sympathy and, indeed, repentance of everyone else to atone for that victimization."[35] Similarly, U.S. Representative William Dannemeyer (Republican, California) has suggested that gay men may have deliberately spread HIV through the blood supply to pressure the government to devote more funds to HIV research and treatment.[36] Although relatively few people believe that HIV disease is a gay plot, such ideas foster stigmatization and even hatred among those who do.

While some conservatives have argued that gays have exaggerated the HIV epidemic to win sympathy, others have argued that the government, to protect the interests of the "gay lobby," has deliberately underestimated both the number of persons already infected with HIV and the ease with which one can become infected. According to Antonio, for example, "There has been a consistent campaign of disinformation about the AIDS virus on the part of many public health officials and the media. Key facts regarding the nature of AIDS, its related conditions and its means of transmission have been glossed over and obscured."[37] Antonio warns his readers that "with the AIDS virus being exuded from almost every bodily orifice, pore and secretion, probably including sweat, prolonged intimate sexual contact of any kind is potentially lethal."[38] He therefore cautions readers against using public toilet seats, expecting condoms to protect them from HIV, sitting on locker room benches, eating in restaurants with gay waiters, and so on.

This social construction of HIV disease as an omnipresent, insidious threat has stimulated right-wing proposals for repressive measures that conservatives assert will stop the spread of HIV. Not so coincidentally, these measures fit into their broader political program. Proposals include quarantining persons with HIV disease, placing restraints on both heterosexual activity and "sodomite promiscuity," and establishing sex education programs that stress the virtues of abstinence and the dangers of homosexuality.[39] The constant calls for such programs both encourage the public to wonder whether persons with HIV disease are too dangerous to live in the community and encourage persons with HIV disease to live in fear of the potential social reactions from others that they may encounter if their illness becomes known.

Racism and the Response to HIV Disease

Because the earliest and so far the majority of persons with HIV disease in the U.S. have been gay men, homophobia has had a major impact on the social construction of the epidemic. However, it is also important to recognize the role played by antagonism toward drug users (who comprise 28 percent of U.S. AIDS cases) and toward nonwhites (who comprise 40 percent of cases, though only 20 percent of the U.S. population).[40]

Explicit prejudice against drug users and nonwhites does not appear as often as prejudice against gays in public statements about HIV disease. Nevertheless, given the continuing racism of many Americans, and in an era of "zero tolerance" for drug use, it seems logical that these attitudes must have contributed to the popular response to HIV disease.

Racism clearly has contributed to the social construction of HIV disease as a disease of the "other." This has been most apparent in the search for the origins of HIV.[41] Although the first cases of HIV disease were diagnosed in the United States, researchers have focused almost solely on Haiti and Africa as possible sources of the virus. This in and of itself suggests a strong willingness among white Americans to believe that people of color somehow foisted HIV on the West. Moreover, most of the suggested theories blame the spread of HIV on non-normative practices. For example, those researchers who suspected a Haitian origin for HIV hypothesized that the virus had spread from animals to humans in Haiti through voodoo rites involving animal sacrifice, and then from Haiti to the U.S. via gay American tourists who supposedly came to Haiti for cheap sex. Thus, not only had Haitians "caused" HIV disease, but they had done so through degenerate and possibly pagan practices.

Other researchers have argued that the virus originated among green monkeys in Central Africa, where HIV seemed to have existed prior to the 1970s. Again, the more responsible writers suggested that African people might have been infected through monkey bites, while the less responsible speculated that Africans had been infected through bestiality or through using monkey glands or blood as aphrodisiacs. Subsequent research strongly suggested that laboratory error had led scientists to overestimate both the rate of HIV infection in Africa before 1970 and the similarity between HIV and the green monkey virus.

These reports suggesting an African origin for HIV have received considerable publicity and have had an impact on the public's image of HIV disease. The British *Sunday Telegraph*, for example, on 21 September 1986 ran a front-page story with the headline "African AIDS Deadly Threat to Britain." The story labelled African tourists and students as the source of AIDS and recommended that British health authorities mandate HIV tests for all resident Africans. This policy was not adopted in Britain but has been adopted elsewhere. In addition, this image of HIV disease as an African illness has led to considerable unofficial discrimination against Africans residing in Europe and Asia.

The Public's Response to HIV Disease

Survey results suggest widespread support for a social construction of HIV disease as a deserved punishment for degenerate "others." Although 87 percent of persons surveyed in a national random sample in late 1987 agreed that "AIDS sufferers should be treated with compassion," and 71 percent disagreed with the statement that "people with AIDS should be isolated from the rest of society," 51 percent agreed that "in general, it's people's own fault if they get AIDS," and 43 percent "sometimes think that AIDS is a punishment for the decline in moral standards."[42] The proportion holding such attitudes remained virtually unchanged between 1985 and 1987.[43] Similarly, one study found that college students consider persons with HIV disease more responsible for their illness than persons with legionnaire's disease or serum hepatitis, even though the latter is spread in the same way as HIV. The students also hold homosexuals more responsible for their illness than heterosexuals, regardless of diagnosis.[44] Such attitudes are common among health care students as well: another study concluded that nursing, medical, and chiropractic students, as well as college students, all considered persons with AIDS less competent and less morally worthy than persons with cancer, diabetes, or heart disease.[45]

The social construction of HIV disease as frightening and mysterious also has found widespread public acceptance. One study found that students would rather share a hospital room with a hepatitis patient than an AIDS patient, even though hepatitis is considerably more infectious than HIV and can be just as deadly.[46] Similarly, another study found that 92 percent of sampled students surveyed would "permit a person dying from cancer to visit the USA for a two-week holiday," but only 66 percent would permit a person with AIDS to do so. In addition, 89 percent would work in an office with someone dying of cancer, but only 50 percent would work with someone who had AIDS.[47]

These attitudes lead many individuals to support restrictive measures against persons with HIV disease. According to a national survey conducted in 1989 by the Los Angeles *Times,* 42 percent of U.S. adults think that some civil liberties must be suspended to stop the spread of AIDS, and only 26 percent say civil liberties must be protected, down from 38 percent in 1987.[48] In the 1987 poll, more than half (52 percent) supported quarantine, one third believed employers should have the right to fire any employees who have AIDS, and 29 percent favored tattooing persons who are infected with HIV.[49] (These questions were not asked in the 1989 poll.) Support for such measures had either remained the same or increased between 1987 and 1985, when the *Times* conducted its first poll on the subject. Yet most public health authorities believe that all these measures would be counterproductive, for they would be exorbitantly expensive, would have to be life-long, and would undoubtedly drive many persons with HIV disease underground, making it more difficult for public health authorities to monitor or control their activities.[50] The 1989 *Times* poll also found that almost three fifths of those interviewed supported compulsory HIV testing for gay men and intravenous drug users, even though most public health authorities agree that testing rarely by itself changes individuals' behavior, leaves people vulnerable to discrimination should they test positive, and does not always produce accurate results.[51]

These attitudes toward persons with HIV disease reflect moral views more than fears of transmission. Several studies suggest that the best way to predict a person's attitudes toward persons with HIV disease is to ask them their attitudes toward gays.[52] Similarly, another study (which did not ask any questions about attitudes toward gays) found that the best way to predict who would support segregating persons with HIV disease was to ask persons if they believed "that America has not recognized the contributions of Christian fundamentalists."[53]

The excessive dread that HIV disease evokes in the public, combined with the belief that HIV disease is somehow deserved, significantly affects the lives of persons with HIV disease. In some cases, they are confronted with these attitudes and the consequences of these attitudes directly, by relatives, friends, doctors, co-workers, and others who choose to castigate or shun them. In other cases, persons with HIV disease are shielded from such responses either because they hide their health status or because their particular associates prove sympathetic. Even in this latter situation, however, they must live with the fear that they will encounter such attitudes and must constantly make choices about whether to hide or reveal the nature of their illness.

The Government's Response

The social construction of HIV disease as a frightening, mysterious disease primarily affecting deserving others has had a significant impact on the government's response to the epidemic and, in turn, on the lives of persons with HIV disease. Because neither the press nor the public displayed much concern about HIV during the early years of the epidemic, conservative politicians (including Presidents Reagan and Bush) have felt free to follow their own bent and to treat HIV disease as a distasteful moral issue rather than as a medical emergency.[54]

In Congress, William Dannemeyer and Jesse Helms have consistently proposed legislation aimed at stopping the spread of HIV by restricting the personal freedom of infected persons. Although

Congress has not yet passed any such laws, some state legislatures have done so. Consequently, fear that such measures will be adopted is a daily fact of life for many persons with HIV disease.

The White House, meanwhile, under Presidents Reagan and Bush, has failed to indicate that HIV disease is a major concern. Rather, its actions consistently have suggested that the illness mostly affects "deserving" gay men. For example, Reagan made no public mention of the epidemic until 1987, when, against the advice of his public health advisors, he called for mandatory HIV testing.[55] Bush's actions differ from Reagan's in stressing that "innocent" babies also can contract HIV disease. His actions, however, suggest no greater sympathy for the vast majority of persons with this illness. The White House's response to the epidemic has both reflected and reinforced the public's willingness to abandon persons with HIV disease to what many consider their deserved fate.

The administration's reluctance to address the epidemic of HIV disease has hindered the country's ability to respond to this crisis. At critical points, it has both restricted the availability of research funds and hampered the development of educational campaigns designed to prevent the spread of HIV. Consequently, many persons have become infected who might otherwise have remained healthy, and many have seen their quality of life deteriorate or have died who might have lived longer, more rewarding lives if the government had made HIV disease a priority from the start.

For several critical, early years, the administration's stance resulted in a serious dearth of funding for research on HIV.[56] According to a major report issued by the Office of Technology Assessment, the Reagan Administration did not ask for any funds for HIV research until 1984.[57] Moreover, for several years, the administration lobbied successfully to keep funding below the level needed for an effective research program. The report documented a pattern of deception by public health administrators who, following orders from their superiors, consistently told Congress that they and the researchers they funded did not need more funds. In fact, many researchers initially did not want to study HIV because they either considered it inconsequential or feared becoming stigmatized as gay if they did so.[58] Others, however, consistently requested funds from administrators, who themselves consistently requested more funds from their superiors. Three years after the Office of Technology Assessment issued its report, the *Report of the Presidential Commission on the Human Immunodeficiency Virus Epidemic* concluded that the government still had not released sufficient funds to develop effective research and education programs.[59]

At first glance, it might seem that the government's dilatory response to the HIV epidemic simply reflected the administration's economic conservatism. The illness first appeared during a period when support for fiscal conservatism had led to widespread budget cuts in health care and biomedical research. Yet the government still managed to respond expeditiously to other health emergencies that arose during the same years. Shilts notes that, for example, "in 1982, the National Institutes of Health's [NIH] research on Toxic Shock Syndrome, a mystery that had by then been solved, amounted to $36,100 per death. NIH Legionnaire's spending in the most recent fiscal year amounted to $34,841 per death. By contrast, the health institute had spent about $3,225 per AIDS death in fiscal 1981 and $8,991 in fiscal 1982. By NIH budget calculations, the life of a gay man was worth about one-quarter that of a member of the American Legion."[60]

Similar figures led Representative Henry Waxman, whose Los Angeles congressional district had been hard hit by the epidemic, to declare during April 1982 hearings before the House of Representatives subcommittee on health and the environment:

> There is no doubt in my mind that if the same disease had appeared among Americans of Norwegian descent, or among tennis players, rather than among gay males, the response of both the government and the medical community would have been different. Legionnaire's disease hit a group of predominantly white, heterosexual, middle-aged members of the American Legion. The respectability of the victims brought

them a degree of attention and funding for research and treatment far greater than that made available so far to the victims of Kaposi's sarcoma. I want to emphasize the contrast, because the more popular Legionnaire's disease affected fewer people and proved less likely to be fatal. What society judged was not the severity of the disease but the social acceptability of the individuals affected with it.

The government's unwillingness to confront the realities of HIV disease also has hindered efforts to stop its spread. At present, and until a cure or vaccine becomes available, educating people about the need to change behaviors that can place them at risk for infection provides the best means to control the spread of HIV. Yet the federal government has proven even less willing to fund public education about HIV than to fund biological research on it.[61]

The few funds that the government has provided have come with many strings attached. These strings make it clear that preventing the spread of HIV is less important to legislators than reaffirming their conservative philosophies and credentials. In 1988, for example, Congress voted to restrict the language that can be used in federally funded education programs regarding HIV disease.[62] Currently, language used in education campaigns directed at specific target groups, such as drug users or gay men, must be language that "would be judged by a reasonable person to be inoffensive to most educated adults *beyond* that group."[63] In other words, brochures designed for distribution to gay men should not offend heterosexuals. The restrictions on audiovisual materials are even tighter, requiring that such materials communicate by "inference rather than by any display of the anogenital area of the body." Consequently, the resulting materials may be too unclear to motivate meaningful behavioral change. The guidelines also state that no federally funded materials shall "promote or encourage, directly, intravenous drug abuse or sexual activity, homosexual or heterosexual." These guidelines effectively prohibit any literature designed to teach people that they can engage in safe sex and still enjoy themselves—a critical gap given that few people will voluntarily give up sex or adopt sexual practices they find unpleasant. Similarly, and even though the majority of American teens are sexually active and a substantial minority experiment with intravenous drugs, in late 1987 the U.S. Senate voted almost unanimously to eliminate funding for *any* HIV education programs for children or young adults that do not emphasize abstinence from sex and drugs, rather than how to engage in these activities safely.[64]

The federal government's unwillingness to fund education about preventing the spread of HIV through drug use has created even greater problems than the lack of funding for education about safer sex.[65] Unlike gay men, drug users do not comprise an organized, politically aware community and cannot expeditiously spread information about the nature or prevention of HIV disease among themselves. At the same time, only a handful of municipalities and no states have proven willing even to experiment with distributing clean needles to drug users or loosening laws regarding the sale and possession of needles. In combination with the lack of educational materials available for drug users, this suggests that the government has decided that drug users are not worth protecting from HIV disease.

The response of the federal government to the epidemic of HIV disease would have been even less productive and more punitive if not for the position taken by the federal courts and by Dr. C. Everett Koop, the surgeon general under former President Reagan. The courts consistently have proven loath to restrict the rights of persons with HIV disease. Throughout the 1970s and into the 1980s, the courts increasingly have recognized the rights of disabled people to work and to get an education. This trend has continued to the present, with the courts in most cases extending the rights of persons with all illnesses and disabilities, including those caused by HIV.[66] Most important, in 1987 the U.S. Supreme Court ruled in *School Board of Nassau Country* v. *Arline* that a teacher with tuberculosis could not be fired unless he or she was unqualified or likely to transmit his or her disease. This ruling seems to apply to persons with AIDS and probably applies to persons with other stages of HIV disease as well. State courts and administrative agencies largely have followed the federal courts' lead and have upheld the rights of workers and students with HIV disease.

Surgeon General Koop also played a critical role in ameliorating the federal government's response to HIV disease. Appointed by President Reagan because of his political conservatism, Koop soon became known for his outspokenness and his unwillingness to let political ideologies (including his own) interfere with the public health measures he considered necessary. Koop continually urged Reagan not to seek repressive actions against persons with HIV disease, and, as much as he could given the constraints imposed on him by the administration, worked to educate the public that HIV is a virus, not a punishment from God. Koop also consistently stressed the need for teaching the public, including children, that the spread of HIV can be prevented even if one chooses to engage in drug use and sexual activity. Koop left the federal government when newly elected President Bush made it clear that he would not be promoted to a Cabinet seat. Whether the federal government will prove any more sympathetic to persons with HIV disease in the 1990s than in the 1980s remains to be seen.

Conclusions

The unique history and biology of HIV disease have led to a social construction of this disease as a terrifying, mysterious "gay disease" that occasionally strikes undeserving (but now suspect), non-gay victims. This definition of HIV disease significantly reduces the quality of life for those who must live with this illness, by affecting both how they are viewed by others and how they view themselves.

The social construction of HIV disease as a deserved punishment has led families to reject their ill relatives, employers to fire employees, friends to abandon friends, and so on. Even persons with HIV disease who have neither had homosexual relationships nor used drugs often find that others reject them on the suspicion that they once did so. Similarly, this social construction has reduced the pressure the government might otherwise have felt to commit substantial resources to research on HIV—research that might have enabled some who are infected to live longer or more meaningful lives. At the same time, this social construction leads to depression and self-hatred among those persons with HIV disease who conclude that they deserved their fate and to bitterness among those who feel they did not.

The social construction of HIV disease as especially mysterious and threatening similarly impairs individuals' lives. Many who do not believe that persons with HIV disease deserve their illness, and who would not shun them on that ground, will shun them because of unrealistic fears of transmission. Moreover, such fears can create tremendous anxiety among those who have the illness about accidentally infecting their loved ones. Similarly, the gaps in scientists' knowledge about the natural history of HIV disease, and the public's confusion about what is known, reinforce both the public's fears of persons with HIV disease and the stress and uncertainty with which those who are infected must live. In sum, the particular horrors that life with HIV brings stem not just from its biology but from its social construction as well.

CHAPTER 3

HIV Disease and the Moral Status of Illness

The social construction of HIV disease often characterizes it as a deserved punishment for immoral behavior. For those who assume that illness is an unchosen, objectively defined, amoral response to infection or genetic conditions, it is difficult to understand how anyone could hold such ideas. In fact, however, social constructions of *all* illnesses develop through subjective, moral judgments that declare ill persons less socially worthy than healthy persons and somehow responsible for their illnesses.

In analyzing the moral status of illness, two key components emerge—blame and dread. *Blame* refers to the idea that ill persons are responsible for their illness, *dread* to the fear of and revulsion against an illness and those who have it. Some illnesses, such as lung cancer among smokers, evoke blame but little dread. Some, such as malaria, evoke dread but little blame. These social definitions set the stage for stigmatizing ill persons. Yet all illnesses are not equally stigmatized, and few are as stigmatized as HIV disease, which evokes both blame and dread. Consequently, to understand the situations of persons with HIV disease, we must understand both the moral status of illness in general and why certain illnesses become especially stigmatized.

Dread and the Moral Status of Illness

At first thought, the dread that healthy persons often feel toward the ill seems simply a logical response, rather than a moral judgment. That healthy persons fear becoming infected by the ill and are repulsed by the aesthetic deterioration that accompanies the physical deterioration of illness seems quite understandable. Underlying these feelings, however, are a series of subjective judgments about the nature of illness. At the most basic level, as Peter Conrad and Joseph Schneider point out, "to define something as a disease or illness is to deem it undesirable"—that is, to make a moral judgment about its value and meaning.[1] It is no surprise that we talk about poverty as an illness but not wealth, obesity but not slenderness, war but not peace. The same process is at work when we describe naturally occurring biological processes or conditions as illnesses. For example, in other societies, osteoporosis, weight gain, and menopause are considered the natural consequences of aging. We, on the other hand, label these conditions illnesses, not because we have some objective biological knowledge about their nature that other societies lack, but because we consider them undesirable.

The moral and political elements in defining illness can become quite explicit. For example, in 1989, the American Society for Plastic and Reconstructive Surgery, the major professional organization for plastic surgeons, officially petitioned the federal Food and Drug Administration to loosen the legal restrictions on the use of breast implants. In their petition, they argued that breast enlargement is medically necessary because "these deformities [i.e., small breasts] are really a disease which in most patients results in feelings of inadequacy, lack of self-confidence, distortion of body image and a total lack of well-being due to a lack of self-perceived femininity."[2] Not surprisingly, others have retorted that this new definition reflects shifting cultural values rather than biological reality.

In the same way that labeling a condition an illness reflects the perceived undesirability of that condition, when we say that someone has an illness or (more strongly) is ill, we judge the desirability of that person. By definition, an ill person is one whose actions, ability, or appearance do not meet social norms. Such a person will automatically be considered less whole and less socially worthy than others. Consequently, they often will evoke irrational fear and revulsion in others, even if they are not held responsible for their conditions. Thus, the dread that illness evokes reflects moral judgments about both the illness itself and the ill person.

Blame and the Moral Status of Illness

Illness, then, refers to biological, psychological, or social conditions considered undesirable by those with the power to create such definitions. Because illness is considered undesirable and because it can strike anyone at any time, it often causes fear and confusion. As a result, people always have tried to explain why illness occurs and, especially, why illness strikes some persons and not others. The resulting explanations relieve individual anxiety by making the world seem less capricious and frightening.

Most often, these explanations define illness as a deserved punishment and blame ill persons for their own illnesses. Such theories provide psychological reassurance by reinforcing people's belief in a "just world" in which only the guilty are punished. Researchers who have studied how people respond to various tragedies, including illness, find that people typically blame the victim to avoid acknowledging that they also might be at risk.[3] Even some ill persons believe that their suffering happened because of their "misdeeds" rather than because of random, impersonal events. Such explanations help make the world comprehensible.

Explaining Illness: Prescientific Ideas

Anthropological studies suggest that such explanations for illness have always been the norm. According to George Foster, all traditional theories of illness causation around the world can be sorted into two somewhat overlapping categories—"personalistic" and "naturalistic."[4] Personalistic theories hold that illness occurs when a god, witch, spirit, or other supernatural power deservedly or maliciously lashes out at an individual. George Murdock reports that most traditional societies, past and present, held or hold such personalistic theories.[5] Naturalistic theories, on the other hand, assert that illness occurs when heat, cold, wind, damp, or other natural events upset the body's equilibrium. Both personalistic and naturalistic theories blame ill persons for causing their illness, whether by displeasing supernatural beings or by exposing themselves to harmful natural elements. And both define ill persons as less morally worthy than others, whether as sinners or as fools.

Personalistic theories played an especially important role in the development of western ideas about illness.[6] In both the Old and the New Testaments, illness is consistently described as divine punishment for sin. For example, Deuteronomy 28 threatens, "If you fail to observe faithfully all the terms of the Teaching that are written in this book, to reverence this honored and awesome name, the Lord our God, the Lord will inflict extraordinary plagues upon you and your offspring, strange and lasting plagues, malignant and chronic diseases. . . . You shall be left a scant few, after having been as numerous as the stars in the skies, because you did not heed the command of the Lord your God." These biblical injunctions are now cited by those who consider HIV disease a divine punishment.

As this quotation suggests, theories connecting illness to sin can be used to explain both illnesses that seem to select certain individuals and those that seem to strike indiscriminately. Bubonic plague, for example, killed between 25 and 50 percent of the population of Europe between the years 1347 and 1351, felling men, women, and children of all ages and classes.[7] At the time, no one knew that plague was caused by a bacterium spread from rats to humans through the bites of infected fleas. Instead, both the public and physicians in Christian Europe believed that this dread illness had appeared because God unleashed disease-causing natural forces, such as "miasma," or air "corrupted" by foul odors and fumes.[8] Because plague struck so widely and randomly, however, theories that explained illness as God's punishment on individual sinners were unconvincing. Instead, most Christians believed plague was a punishment from God for the sins of humanity as a whole. Whether one lived or died, then, was a matter of mercy or luck, rather than a marker of individual guilt or innocence. Muslim theologians, on the other hand, who did not share the Christian emphasis on sin, hell, and the apocalypse, defined plague as a divine punishment for infidels who rejected Allah, but "a mercy and a martyrdom from God for the faithful Muslim."[9] They believed that Muslims who died from plague, like persons who died in holy wars, were guaranteed a place in paradise.[10] In both Muslim and Christian countries, therefore, although persons who had plague were often dreaded and shunned because of fear of contagion, their illness was not considered a sign of personal sin or blame and did not lead to religious or moral sanctions against them.

In contrast, the history of leprosy demonstrates the substantial consequences for individuals when illness is attributed to personal sin. Because of its ability to ravage individuals' appearance—especially the face and hands (parts considered most representative of persons' true beings)—leprosy was always a dreaded disease. In addition, more than any other illness in premodern times, it evoked accusations of blame. Although the Old and New Testaments consistently describe illness as punishment for sin (except in the book of Job), leprosy stands out because it is so often specifically named as the consequence of an individual's sin.[11] This explanation for leprosy, coupled perhaps with some sense that leprosy was contagious, led biblical society to isolate affected individuals in every possible way. Leviticus 13 orders, "As for the person with a leprous affection, his clothes shall be rent, his head shall be left bare, and he shall cover over his upper lip; and he shall call out, 'Unclean! Unclean!' . . . Being unclean, he shall dwell apart; his dwelling shall be outside the camp."

This approach continued essentially unchanged for centuries.

Throughout the Middle Ages and until the Reformation, for example, persons with leprosy were banished formally from all social intercourse, through a version of the mass for the dead known as the "lepers' mass." Following the mass, a priest would shovel dirt on the individual's feet to symbolize his or her civil and religious death and then formally forbid the individual ever to enter any church, market, or other gathering place. [12] The person with leprosy was also forbidden to wash in any springs or streams, to drink from another's cup, to wear anything other than the special "leper's dress," to touch anything before buying it, to talk to anyone without first moving downwind, to touch any infant or child, and so on. This social banishment continued even after death, for persons with leprosy, like suicides and others who committed mortal sins, could not be buried in sanctified ground.

Following the Enlightenment, religious ideas about illness began to lose their influence in the western world. Yet ill people continued to be blamed for their illnesses. Many members of the public could accept, for example, that polio or scarlet fever were caused by microorganisms, but continued to believe that leprosy, epilepsy, and syphilis were divine punishments. Each of these latter illnesses had been popularly linked to sin for centuries, and it would take time before the modest growth in scientific knowledge could overcome these ideas. For example, for decades after 1872, when Dr. Gerhard Hansen demonstrated that leprosy was caused by a bacterium, the government continued to turn over most of the care for persons with leprosy to nuns and priests rather than doctors and nurses, reflecting and reinforcing the idea that leprosy was a problems of morals rather than medicine. [13] Similarly, even after it became clear that leprosy is extremely difficult to transmit, the dread and blame attached to leprosy remained strong, and the treatment of persons with leprosy remained far harsher than that of others with far more contagious illnesses. For much of this century, U.S. leprosaria resembled prisons more than hospitals. [14] Persons sent to these leprosaria could be kept involuntarily for life. They were physically separated from their families, encouraged to change their names to protect their families from disgrace, and sometimes advised to let their families believe they had died rather than expose them to the stigma of having a relative with leprosy.[15] They also were denied the right to vote, to marry, or even to use a telephone—actions that suggest the government feared moral as well as physical contagion.

The present-day response to HIV disease suggests the continuing strength of ideas linking illness and immorality. Even when individuals do not blame ill persons on moral grounds, however, they may blame them for other reasons. Cholera, for example, was one of the most feared illnesses to appear in the post-Enlightenment period, and in some ways the illness most like HIV disease.[16] Like HIV disease, cholera was particularly dreaded because it was a new illness for westerners, first appearing outside of Asia in about 1830. And like HIV disease, the death rates were high, averaging 50 percent but ranging as high as 90 percent of those infected. Moreover, cholera killed suddenly and spectacularly, its victims dying of overwhelming dehydration brought on by uncontrollable diarrhea and vomiting.

We now know that cholera is caused by a waterborne bacterium, generally transmitted when human wastes contaminate food or drinking water. Because of the connection between cholera and sanitation problems, it more often strikes poor people than rich. To be plausible, therefore, any theory of cholera had to explain why the poor were more susceptible.

At the time cholera struck the West, the germ theory of illness had not yet won acceptance (and would not for another forty or fifty years). However, ideas about the nature of illness had changed considerably, as people increasingly accepted that scientific principles controlled the natural order. Although theories that linked illness to divine will still influenced popular opinion, the new "scientific" thinking posited that illness occurred when biological forces combined with personal susceptibility. Doctors argued that illness occurred when persons whose constitutions either were naturally weak or had been weakened by unhealthy behaviors came in

contact with dangerous miasma. According to this theory, therefore, individuals became ill not because their behavior was immoral
but simply because it was unhealthy.

On the surface, this new theory seems more rational and less
moralistic than previous ones. In fact, however, it reinforced moral
judgments against ill persons, because physicians asserted that cholera attacked individuals who had weakened their constitutions
through improper lifestyles.[17] The poor, they argued, had caused
their own illnesses, first by lacking the initiative required to escape
poverty and then by choosing to eat an unhealthy diet, live in dirty
conditions, or drink too much alcohol. Thus, for example, the New
York City Medical Council could conclude in 1832 that "the disease in the city is confined to the imprudent, the intemperate, and
to those who injure themselves by taking improper medicines."[18]
The wealthy, on the other hand, would generally become ill only
if they were gluttonous or greedy, or if they "innocently" had the
misfortune to inhale some particularly noxious air.

Using this theory, doctors, foreshadowing what has happened
with HIV disease, divided patients into the "guilty" (the overwhelming majority), the "innocent," and the "suspect," and hospitals provided or refused care accordingly.[19] This theory of illness
allowed the upper classes to adopt the new, scientific explanations
for illness while retaining older, moralistic assumptions about ill
people and avoiding any sense of responsibility for alleviating the
plight of the poor or ill. Thus instead of believing that immorality
led directly to illness, people now believed that immorality left one
susceptible to the biological forces that led to illness.

Modern Theories of Illness

Despite the tremendous growth in medical knowledge about
illness in the last century, popular explanations for illness have remained remarkably stable. Theories connecting illness to sin continue to appear, as do theories that conceptualize illness as a direct
consequence of poorly chosen and hence irresponsible (although not
necessarily sinful) behavior.[20] For example, although most persons

in the developed nations know that influenza and the common cold are caused by viruses, most continue to hold essentially naturalistic theories of illness—warning their children to eat warm foods, dress warmly in cold weather, and cover up against the rain to avoid illness. One English study of patients' ideas about colds concluded:

> There is the strong implication of personal responsibility for the condition, which has been caused by one's own careless-ness, stupidity or lack of foresight. You get a cold when you "don't dress properly," "go outside after washing your hair," "allow your head to get wet," "walk barefoot on a cold floor," "wash your hair when you don't feel well," and so on. . . . If, despite adequate precautions such as proper clothing, and so on, one still got a cold, it was still your responsibility.[21]

Similarly, many people now blame illness on individual life-style. This conception of illness has become popular in recent years among both the mass media and public health authorities.[22] Maga-zines are filled with articles on subjects such as self-healing and "superimmunity"; they exhort individuals to protect or restore their health through diet, exercise, stress reduction, and the like.[23] Si-multaneously, the government—even while it continues to subsi-dize the tobacco and beef industries—has invested substantial resources in education campaigns to encourage the public to stop smoking and to eat a healthier diet.

Another popular ideology ties illness not to individual actions but to individual personalities.[24] For example, nineteenth-century Americans generally believed that persons developed tuberculosis (one of the most widespread and feared diseases of that epoch) be-cause they "burned" with the fevers of thwarted passions. As tuber-culosis came under control and cancer replaced it in the popular imagination as the most dreaded illness, the image of a cancer-prone personality developed. For example, some recent newspaper accounts of actress Gilda Radner's losing battle against cancer highlighted the role her personality played in her illness. According to one article, "Joanna Bull of the Wellness Community in Santa Monica, . . . an inspirational force in Radner's battle to lick the odds, remembers that 'Gilda always had this wonderful will to live. Yet she also exhibited the same preconditioning virtually all [cancer patients] have. Fear. Hopelessness. Negativity. What the Wellness Community is all about, and what Gilda came to appreciate, is that a positive outlook can improve the quality of life—up to and including the immune system.' "[25] Similarly, and despite recent studies refuting this theory, the media continue to assume that persons with "type A" personalities are more likely to suffer heart attacks.[26]

Others, meanwhile, have argued that illness occurs not because individuals ignore their bodies or have illness-producing personalities, but because they *choose* to become ill. The most influential statement of this theory appears in the book *Love, Medicine and Miracles* by surgeon Bernie Siegel, which has sold more than 1.5 million copies.[27] Siegel postulates that people become ill because they "need" their illness—to escape a stressful work situation, receive sympathy from their spouses, punish themselves for misdeeds, or for some other reason. The underlying principle, according to Siegel, is that people become susceptible to illness when they do not love themselves enough to take care of their emotional needs. Thus, he suggests, although ill persons should not abandon orthodox medicine, medicine can only help superficially, for they will only find lasting cures when they truly desire a healthy, long life.

The theories of Bernie Siegel and others affect the way the healthy view the ill, as well as how ill persons view themselves. Clearly, individual factors such as stress, personality, and lifestyle can affect individual susceptibility to illness. Yet by focusing on these factors as the primary or sole source of illness, these theories suggest that individuals are the main cause of their illnesses. As a result, these theories can encourage others, including health care providers, to stigmatize and reject ill persons. In addition, by emphasizing how individuals trigger biological responses, they encourage policymakers to ignore how social and environmental factors combine with biological factors to promote illness.[28] For example, magazines and books that emphasize how individuals make themselves ill rarely discuss how factors largely beyond individual control, such as poverty, malnutrition, pollution, or unsafe conditions in our houses, cars, or workplaces, can produce ill health. Nor do they discuss how social factors pressure individuals to adopt less-than-healthy lifestyles—how unemployed teenagers with poor job prospects may smoke cigarettes to demonstrate their adulthood, or how young mothers who lack assistance with child care may not have time for the recommended three sessions per week of aerobic exercise, or how workers may suffer injuries because of unsafe equipment rather than because of their carelessness. As Barbara Katz Rothman notes:

> Think of the anti-smoking, anti-drinking "behave yourself" campaigns aimed increasingly at pregnant women. What are the causes [as identified in these campaigns] of prematurity, fetal defects, damaged newborns—flawed products? Bad mothers, of course—inept workers. One New York City subway ad series shows two newborn footprints, one from a full-term and one from a premature infant. The ads read, "Guess which baby's mother smoked while pregnant?" Another asks "Guess which baby's mother drank while pregnant?" And yet another: "Guess which baby's mother didn't get prenatal care?" I look in vain for the ad that says "Guess which baby's mother tried to get by on welfare?"; "Guess which baby's mother had to live on the streets?"; or "Guess which baby's mother was beaten by her husband?"[29]

In sum, theories of illness that focus on individual responsibility reinforce the status quo and rationalize societal rejection and maltreatment of, or indifference toward, the ill.

Stigmatized Illnesses

Inherent in the social response to illness is the idea that the ill are less socially worthy than the healthy and that ill persons are somehow responsible for their own illness, whether because of sin, unhealthy behavior, or illness-causing personality. As a result, the well may feel justified in stigmatizing the ill, ignoring their needs, and maintaining social structures that unintentionally promote illness.

All illnesses do not provoke equally strong responses, however. To understand the situation faced by persons with HIV disease, therefore, we have to understand not only the general processes involved in responses to illness but also how, why, and with what consequences some illnesses are set apart from others as especially terrible and especially worthy of stigma.

Illnesses will result in the greatest stigma when the blame and dread they evoke are strongest. This occurs when six conditions are met.

First, blame, dread, and hence stigma will be greatest when illnesses are connected to already stigmatized groups.[30] The response to HIV disease amply demonstrates this process. Initially identified in marginal populations (gay men, drug users, and black Haitian immigrants), HIV disease was and is considered a fitting punishment for those who are known or assumed to engage in stigmatized activities. HIV disease now can be found in people from the mainstream of American life—heterosexual, non-drug-using, white middle-class men and women. Instead of the stigma of the illness lessening, however, that stigma has encompassed many of these additional individuals and made their pasts suspect, as friends and neighbors wonder what they did to contract this illness. Similarly, when cholera first struck the United States, it produced especially great fear and revulsion because it was considered a vile, Asian disease by white Americans, most of whom considered Asians inherently inferior. Moreover, cholera in the U.S. disproportionately struck poor Irish immigrants, whom nativist Americans considered only slightly better than Asians. As a result, racist and nativist sentiment contributed to the dread with which cholera and its victims were viewed and to the belief that those who fell ill were somehow responsible for their own illness. In contrast, despite great public fear of polio, infected persons were pitied more than shunned because they were predominantly children and were often from middle- or upper-class homes.

Second, illnesses are likely to be especially stigmatized if they are linked to sexuality—and are especially likely to be linked to sexuality if they are stigmatized. Because western attitudes toward sexuality are ambivalent at best, many members of the public are especially repulsed by illnesses that serve as markers for sexual activity, particularly if that activity is considered stigmatized.[31] For example, in the past, many people believed that cancer and leprosy were caused by either sexual immorality or sexual repression.[32] This idea both reflected and contributed to the dread with which these illnesses were viewed. Similarly, to reduce the stigma their patients would experience, nineteenth-century doctors sometimes declared that their patients had contracted gonorrhea from door knobs or toilet seats. The stigma of gonorrhea increased substantially once it became clear that it could only be transmitted to adults through sexual activity.[33]

Fear as well as revulsion makes illnesses linked to sexuality especially stigmatized. Despite western culture's ambivalence toward sexuality, sexual drives remain a basic part of human nature. As a result, fear is especially high whenever an illness threatens the ability to act on one's sexual desires. Sexually transmitted illnesses (such as HIV disease, syphilis, and gonorrhea) can directly or indirectly limit individuals' sexual repertoires, either by diminishing physical capabilities or by forcing them to adopt less satisfying sexual routines to protect their or their partners' health. In addition, all sexually transmitted diseases can psychologically affect sexual ability by causing people to identify sex with pain, illness, and even death. Sexual ability also may decrease if ill persons feel personally polluted, worry about sexual rejection, or fear they will infect others.

Third, illnesses are also likely to be especially stigmatized if no vaccine is available and, accurately or inaccurately, they are believed to be contagious.[34] For example, leprosy, which had once been endemic throughout Europe, vanished almost entirely from that continent by the sixteenth century and never became a significant problem in North America except among immigrants from tropical areas.[35] As a result, most western scientists hypothesized that leprosy was a hereditary Asian illness to which westerners were immune. Consequently, popular fear of leprosy declined substantially. These fears only returned in the late nineteenth century, when scientists proved that leprosy was contagious; the death of the well-know missionary, Father Damien, proved that Europeans were not immune; and epidemiologists suggested that imported black, East Indian, and Chinese laborers were spreading leprosy in the New World.

Fourth, illnesses will result in especially great stigma if they create visible, disfiguring, dehumanizing changes that seem to transform the person into something beastly or alien.[36] The rotting hands and noses of persons with leprosy, the uncontrollable writhing of epileptic seizures, the purple lesions of Kaposi's sarcoma, or the dementia of end-stage AIDS produce a horror that the crutches and withered legs of someone with polio cannot. In contrast, nineteenth-century writers could consider tuberculosis romantic because its symptoms mirrored the pale fragility to which Victorian women and aesthetic men aspired.[37]

Fifth, illnesses will be especially stigmatized if they are "consequential," producing death or extensive disability and appearing to threaten not just scattered individuals but society as a whole.[38] HIV disease, for example, has evoked especially strong dread because it causes progressive disability, seems uniformly fatal, continues to spread, and is expected to have a significant impact on economic and social life. In contrast, despite the fact that at least

21 million people were killed by the influenza epidemic of 1918, that epidemic generated relatively mild responses among the public.[39] Because it appeared during World War I, the newspapers were too preoccupied to pay it much attention. This lack of coverage, combined with the daily reports of war horrors, made the epidemic seem relatively inconsequential. Moreover, only a small percentage of those who became ill died, those who survived did not experience any lingering disabilities, and the epidemic ended in a matter of months.

Sixth, illnesses will be especially stigmatized if mysteries remain regarding their natural history, producing an "uncertain certainty," in which the public knows that it does *not* know critical facts about how the illness is spread, what its effects will be, and who will become ill next.[40] For example, HIV disease now and cholera in the past created tremendous dread in part because they were newly discovered illnesses about which the public had many unanswered questions. We still do not know, for example, exactly how long people may be infected with HIV before developing symptoms or whether all who are infected with the virus will die eventually. In contrast, there was nothing mysterious about the 1918 influenza epidemic. Although the particular strain of influenza involved was unusually virulent, neither doctors nor patients had any doubt about its nature or meaning.

The Moral Status of HIV Disease

To an extent greater than any other modern illness, HIV disease is stigmatized. The connection between HIV disease, already stigmatized groups, and sexuality, combined with the fear generated by this contagious, incurable, disfiguring illness that many people still consider mysterious and incomprehensible, combine to evoke both blame and dread on a level far beyond that evoked by other modern illnesses.

To some extent, as HIV disease spreads to what is still referred to as the "general population," we may find that persons with HIV disease are less often blamed for causing their illness through their sins. At the same time, however, the tendency to find more secular reasons for blaming persons with HIV disease seems to be growing, as philosophies linking illness to personality and personal choices gain acceptance.

Along these lines, several books are now available on avoiding or curing HIV disease through improving your immune system. These books include *AIDS: Passageway to Transformation* and *Psychoimmunity and the Healing Process: A Holistic Approach to Immunity and Aids.*[41]

The most influential of these works is *The AIDS Book: Creating a Positive Approach,* by Louise Hay.[42] In that book, Hay extends Bernie Siegel's analysis and argues that HIV disease exists because people do not love themselves or others enough. She refers to HIV disease consistently as a "dis-ease," to reinforce the idea that it is an emotional more than a physical illness. Hay's works are so popular that they now comprise an entire cottage industry; one can get books, audiotapes, and videotapes from Hay describing her philosophy and how to implement it. Her Wednesday night "Hay rides" in Los Angeles attract approximately eight hundred people every week, and her lecture tours routinely sell out.

Although Hay accepts the dominant medical paradigm regarding the nature of HIV and encourages persons with HIV disease to continue standard medical treatment, she proposes a distinctly nonmedical view about why people become infected:

> I believe that we are all exposed to everything [germs or viruses] that is floating by. . . . I believe that what we pick up depends on where we are in consciousness. That is, "What do we believe about life and about ourselves?" Do we believe that "life is hard and we always get the short end of the stick" or that "life is full of war and hate" so that we are open to all illnesses, or "I'm no good anyway, so what difference does it make" or "I've always known I would die young." If our

beliefs run along these lines, then our immune systems will be lowered, and we will be free to catch the "popular" disease of the moment. If our immune systems are strong and healthy, then our bodies will automatically fight off whatever dis-ease may pass our way.[43]

She uses a similar argument to explain why HIV disease has struck some groups more than others:

It is interesting that the first people to be affected with the dis-ease AIDS are those who are oppressed or feel unable to fend for themselves—Africans, Haitians, gays, hemophiliacs, drug users, people getting blood transfusions, and the babies of people in these groups. These are mostly people with lots of unexpressed anger and rage towards their families or towards society as a whole. These feelings may be combined with feelings of helplessness and hopelessness to make any positive changes in their lives. They are not yet aware of the power of their own minds.[44]

This reasoning allows Hay to explain an inherently sociological problem (why persons who experience oppression become ill more often than others) in strictly psychological terms.

Extrapolating from this, Hay encourages those who want to end illness to try to change individual behaviors and attitudes, rather than changing social conditions. Hay's advice for both the infected and the uninfected is to create personal psychological changes that will enable one to live "from your highest level" and "experience unconditional love."[45] She argues that HIV disease can be cured if these and other actions are taken early enough, and provides examples of clients she believes have cured themselves through nutrition, meditation, visualization exercises (such as imagining their immune system as soldiers fighting disease), and affirmations (such as telling themselves that they are strong or that they love their body and want it to heal).

Hay has developed a large following among persons with HIV

disease because she offers them a sense that they can control their destinies. As a result, she undoubtedly has improved the quality of life for many persons in the early stages of HIV disease, when her ideas seem most plausible and provide a sense of hope. However, if curing oneself represents a victory in Hay's philosophy, then succumbing to illness becomes a defeat. As a result, as the illness inevitably progresses, those persons with HIV disease who adopt this philosophy may find that this sense of hope and personal power degenerates into a sense of failure.[46]

Conclusions

In sum, throughout history social constructions of illnesses have involved moral judgments. From biblical descriptions of lepers' "sins" to modern descriptions of the "cancer-prone" personality, these social constructions have encouraged the healthy to dread the ill and to blame them for their fates. Yet although blame and dread are key components in our responses to all illnesses, the extent to which they are evoked varies from illness to illness. HIV disease has become an especially stigmatized illness because of the especially strong blame and dread it generates; it is an illness that is connected to already stigmatized groups and to sexuality. It is incurable, contagious, disfiguring, consequential, and still somewhat mysterious. New theories of HIV disease that locate its cause in individual personalities rather than behavior cannot eliminate the tendency to blame the ill but can only create new reasons for doing so.

Thus, from the time of diagnosis, persons with HIV disease confront not only the actual and potential physical devastation that their illness can wreak, but also social constructions that encourage blame and dread in themselves and others. The next four chapters examine how the social construction and the biology of HIV disease affect the lives of those who have this illness and explore how they cope with these threats to their lives and self-images.

CHAPTER 4

Becoming a Person
with HIV Disease

In biological terms, becoming a person with HIV disease requires only that one become infected with HIV. In sociological terms, however, it requires not only that one become infected but also that one recognize this change and reevaluate him- or herself accordingly. That reevaluation requires individuals to deal with three tasks: assessing one's risk of infection and the meaning of any symptoms one exhibits before diagnosis, obtaining a diagnosis, and, after diagnosis, conceptualizing the consequences of HIV disease for one's future.

Assessing the Risk of HIV Disease

For many individuals, the first step in becoming persons with HIV disease is recognizing that they are at risk. Because of the various ways HIV can be transmitted, however, this recognition comes sooner to some than to others. HIV disease was first described in the medical literature in June 1981 as a new and deadly disease that apparently affected only gay men. Gay newspapers and magazines, especially the *Advocate* and the *New York Native,* began covering the story immediately. Two months later, a group of gay men living in New York City founded an organization known as Gay Men's

Health Crisis to promote education and research about HIV disease. Surveys conducted in Chicago, New York, and San Francisco suggest that as early as 1983, and at least in those three cities, most gay men knew how HIV was transmitted and that they were at risk.[1]

Other groups have taken somewhat longer to realize that they are at risk. In 1982, the CDC announced that drug users, persons who had received blood transfusions in the last few years, and hemophiliacs were at risk for HIV disease; in 1983 it announced that heterosexual partners of infected persons were at risk. As early as 1984, drug users surveyed in New York City and New Jersey knew that they could contract HIV disease if they shared needles;[2] probably, however, the farther users lived from the cities where HIV first struck the longer they took to learn this. By 1985, almost all persons interviewed in national polls knew that HIV could be transmitted through heterosexual and homosexual contact, blood transfusions, and shared needles.[3]

Because this knowledge is so widespread in the gay male community, HIV disease plays a large role in the thoughts of gay and bisexual men. Several men I interviewed had assumed they were infected long before they were diagnosed. The rest had experienced long months of anxiety about whether they would become ill, for although they could change their behavior to protect themselves against future infection, they could not retroactively eliminate any past exposure to the virus.

In contrast, half the women I interviewed did not learn that they were at risk until after they were diagnosed. Two did not know of their husband's or lover's drug use or affairs. Two did not know that blood transfusions could transmit HIV. One did not know that intravenous needles could transmit HIV. One (married to a hemophiliac) did not know that hemophiliacs were at risk. And one, who had divorced her drug-using husband ten years before, had assumed that she was not infected because she had stayed healthy for so many years after leaving him.

Moreover, of the seven women who knew they were at risk,

only the two who still used intravenous drugs at the time of diagnosis had worried about contracting HIV disease. Four of the remaining five assumed their risk was small because they had stopped using drugs several years earlier. The fifth simply had ignored the possibility that a former lover who had hemophilia might have infected her.

For those who either do not know or refuse to believe they are at risk, HIV disease is not an emotional problem until symptoms start appearing. For the rest, however, uncertainty about whether they will develop HIV disease is a major source of stress, and coping with uncertainty a critical task. At this point, then, persons with HIV disease must begin developing the skills that will help them deal with this and all the other uncertainties they will face in the coming months, as they try to understand what has happened to their lives and their futures.

Uncertainty is a central concern for all chronically and terminally ill persons and a major source of stress in their lives.[4] To deal with uncertainty, individuals must develop cognitive frameworks that help them understand their situations and thus help them feel that they can predict the outcomes of their actions. To cope with uncertainty about whether they will develop HIV disease, and before their own health deteriorates, individuals can construct theories that explain why, despite their behaviors, they are not really at risk. These theories typically suggest that HIV disease attacks only physically weak persons who "promiscuously" share their bodies or their needles with foolishly chosen partners and who live in areas where HIV disease is widespread. For example, Carol, a twenty-five-year-old housewife and mother who lives in a working-class Phoenix suburb, had started injecting cocaine in 1984. In 1986, she learned that drug users were at risk for HIV disease. Nevertheless, she had concluded that her risk of infection was slight. As she explains, "The person that I got it from was the only person I used drugs with. . . . It wasn't like I went down to a shooting gallery in South Phoenix [a poor, minority neighborhood] and just picked needles up off the ground." Similarly, Daryl, a Phoenix stockbroker in his early thirties, explains that although he and his friends had worried about HIV disease, they had not used condoms because they had convinced themselves that "there's only nine people in Arizona who have it and four of them are dead and two of them live in Tucson. So what are your chances? Even though we knew about it and we knew how awful it was, it was like, no, that's something that happens someplace else, not in Phoenix."

As more cases of HIV disease appeared, however, and as the individuals themselves began developing health problems, these theories provided less comfort. This was especially true for the fourteen men and women who had seen friends, lovers, or spouses sicken or die. As a result, some individuals alternately denied and brooded on the risks they had taken—emotionally unable to accept the fact that they might die from a dread disease yet intellectually unable fully to reject the possibility. For example, Calvin, a forty-one-year-old store manager, had both used intravenous drugs and engaged in extensive homosexual activity. As a result, he had every reason to suspect he might be infected. Moreover, one of his close friends had been among the first persons in Phoenix diagnosed with HIV disease, so Calvin knew that the disease had reached Arizona. Yet note how Calvin shifts in a matter of moments from describing how he believed he was immune to describing how his fear of contracting HIV disease had kept him awake nights:

Q: Before you had symptoms, were you hearing about AIDS? Were people worrying about it?

A: Yeah. I've been aware of AIDS since it first was discovered in '82, but I chose not to listen simply because it was too frightening and I thought it would never happen to me. . . . I heard about the dos and don'ts—sexually, what was safe and what wasn't safe, IV drug use—all those things the gay community could be prone to get involved in. But I chose to not listen simply because I felt it would never happen to me. . . .

Q: Had you worried about getting AIDS?

A: Yeah. It had frightened me when it first came out and there were many nights that I lost sleep. . . . So I worried about it. It was like a paranoia.

The Decision to Test for HIV

Since mid 1985, people who wonder if they will get HIV disease have been able to eliminate some of their uncertainty about the future by taking an ELISA test. This test ascertains if an individual has been infected with HIV. For those who test negative (that is, uninfected), the ELISA test can virtually eliminate uncertainty about their health status. Those who test positive, however, merely trade one form of uncertainty for another, because the test cannot determine how soon, or even if, they will develop health problems associated with HIV disease. As a result, a positive test result can significantly increase anxiety.[5] In addition, a positive test by itself can result in stigma if it becomes known, even if the individual has no health problems. For these reasons, in the first years after the test was developed, most gay community leaders warned against testing.[6] Only after about 1988, when promising treatments became available to those who could document that they were infected with HIV, did these leaders change their position. The effect was felt immediately; Siegel and her colleagues report that a substantial proportion of the gay men living in New York City whom they interviewed in 1988 and 1989 had avoided testing in previous years because they feared discrimination but had subsequently gotten tested so that, should they test positive, they could obtain prophylactic medical care.[7] In the future, therefore, more individuals will know they are infected before symptoms appear, as the move toward earlier testing spreads across the nation.

In part because of these warnings from gay leaders, all but two of the men I interviewed in 1986 and 1987 had decided that they would feel more in control of their destinies by refusing to obtain such ambiguous knowledge.[8] Chris, for example, is a twenty-eight-year-old construction worker who describes himself as "addicted" to sex and alcohol. Despite (or perhaps because of) his many previous sexual contacts and his worsening health, he had decided not to get tested. As he explains, "I figured if I was tested and tested positive, I'd worry myself into coming down with it, because I have great fantasies with anything that starts to bother me. I just blow it out of proportion. And so I decided against it. . . . If I came down with it, I came down with it, and I'd have to worry about it then." Chris, like almost all the other men, eventually got tested only to confirm his diagnosis once his symptoms became unavoidably obvious and disabling.

In contrast, the women proved far more willing to get tested at earlier stages of HIV disease. Ten of the fourteen sought testing before any symptoms appeared. Of these fourteen, three sought testing as soon as they learned that they were at risk and that a test existed. Another three sought testing once their sense of risk moved from abstract to concrete, when they learned that a sexual or needle-sharing partner had HIV disease. Three were pressured to take the test by their lovers and one was tested as a condition of employment.

In large measure, the women sought testing sooner than the men because their fears of infecting others were greater and their fears of the test were less. Unlike gay men, who can argue that their sexual partners are already at risk, the women typically believe that they are the only potential source of infection for their husbands or lovers. As a result, they felt ethically obligated, or had been required by their lovers, to get tested to protect others. Also, unlike gay men who live in a community at risk in which the possible dangers of the test have been widely discussed, the women only learned of its social and psychological dangers after they were tested. As a result, they had had no reason to avoid getting tested.

Carrie's situation illustrates a very different route to testing than that of the others I interviewed, for Carrie never chose to be tested. A career military officer, she was tested by the military as part of its routine, yearly testing of all soldiers. Many gay male soldiers have responded to mandatory testing by resigning from the military. Most of the rest have chosen to get tested privately before the military tests them. If they learn that they are infected, they resign quietly to avoid a dishonorable discharge. As far as she knew, however, Carrie had no reason to fear the test. She had experienced no health symptoms and knew of no lover or ex-lover who was bisexual or a drug user. Only after she tested positive did she learn that an ex-lover had used drugs. Although Carrie is the only person I interviewed who learned of her infection with HIV in this way, her situation will become increasingly common, if the trend toward testing prisoners, hospital patients, pregnant women, and the like continues.

As mandatory testing and voluntary but routine testing spread, and as the development of new drugs motivates individuals to get tested, a greater number and variety of people will get tested earlier in the course of the disease. Getting tested, however, does not guarantee that one will learn whether one is infected, for current tests are not perfect. Individuals who test negative are routinely told to test again in a few months to eliminate the possibility that they have been infected but have not yet developed enough antibodies to HIV for the test to detect. Nor is a positive test necessarily conclusive, as Grace's story illustrates.

Grace, a thirty-two-year-old mother and office worker, was tested for HIV as a routine precaution at the request of a new lover. She had not exhibited any symptoms of HIV disease, and her only source of risk was her drug-using ex-husband, whom she had divorced ten years earlier. To her surprise, she tested positive on the ELISA test. Because this test was designed to protect the nation's blood supply from contamination with HIV, it was designed so that contaminated blood would rarely escape detection (that is, so that there would be very few false negatives). Any test that produces few false negatives, however, will produce considerably more false positives, indicating inaccurately that individuals are infected with

HIV. The test is especially likely to have this effect among populations, like white women, in which infection is rare. As a result, whenever a patient tests positive on the ELISA, most doctors automatically will repeat the test. If the second test is also positive, doctors will then administer the more accurate (and more expensive) Western Blot test. In Grace's case, two ELISAs came back positive and two subsequent Western Blot tests came back "indeterminate," the results insufficient to identify whether she is infected with HIV. She reports, "I found it very confusing. It made me crazy actually trying to figure it out." A county health officer from the testing facility told her that some people, most of whom are really negative, test indeterminate all their lives—a situation Grace believes "would be a really crummy way to live." Since then, she has twice tested negative on the ELISA but continues to test indeterminate on the Western Blot.

Although Grace is the only person I interviewed who is in this amorphous position, her situation is becoming more common. As the ELISA test increasingly is used on persons at low risk for HIV disease, false positives and indeterminate test results will become increasingly common. Such results are especially common among women. During pregnancy, the body has to learn not to reject the fetus even though it is a "foreign" object. As a result, women who are or have been pregnant, like persons with immune system disorders, lose some of their ability to recognize viral infections. Because of this similarity in blood chemistry between currently or formerly pregnant women and persons with immune disorders, such women are more likely than other persons to inaccurately be labeled HIV-positive. Yet despite this danger, some doctors are now calling for routine HIV testing during prenatal care; the American College of Obstetricians and Gynecologists recommends routine HIV testing for all women considered at risk for HIV as well as all women living in areas where HIV is relatively common.[9] Consequently, the number of women who, like Grace, may have to endure months or even years of uncertainty about whether they are infected with HIV may grow substantially.

Interpreting Symptoms and Seeking Diagnoses

The initial symptoms of HIV disease can take many forms, including rashes, fevers, night sweats, weight loss, diarrhea, tiredness, difficulty breathing, and swollen lymph nodes. Once symptoms begin to appear, individuals must decide how to interpret them and how to respond.

The problems involved in making these decisions differ depending on whether or not individuals know they are or might be infected with HIV. Those who know have readily available explanations for any symptoms that appear. Yet they still must wonder if these symptoms are a result of HIV disease or of some unrelated health problems. Carol, for example, even though asymptomatic, was tested for HIV once she learned that the one person she occasionally shared needles with had been diagnosed with HIV disease. Her ambiguous health status causes her constant stress:

> That's the things that are aggravating to me about living with the HIV and just wondering day to day when is it going to progress to the next stage. Every time I have a headache, every time I can't remember something quite right, I wonder is it the stress and all the bullshit that's going on [in my life] or, my God, is this going into the second stage? And then how quick will it go into AIDS after it's gone into the second stage? That's something you live with day to day. Every little thing. I'll get a sore throat and think, "Oh, it's in my lymph nodes." You know and you start feeling around. It's just, it's scary. [It's] something that never goes away.

The appearance of symptoms presents a different set of problems for those who do not know they are infected with HIV. Because symptoms generally build gradually, persons with HIV disease at first can accommodate to them. As a result, they, like persons who develop other chronic illnesses, initially may explain their symptoms using preexisting cognitive frameworks that minimize the symptoms' importance.[10] Several blamed their night sweats and exhaustion on the Arizona heat. Others confused the symptoms of HIV disease with the side effects of drug use or drug withdrawal, both of which can cause weight loss, sweating, and diarrhea. Although these theories eventually proved wrong, in the interim they reduced uncertainty and hence stress by allowing individuals to feel they understood what was happening to them.

Although some individuals minimized their symptoms out of ignorance, most appeared consciously or unconsciously to downplay their symptoms because they preferred to maintain unrealistic theories about their health rather than to obtain accurate but depressing knowledge. Compared to the other people I interviewed, Kevin, a twenty-three-year-old sales clerk, seems far more overwhelmed by his illness, unable to cope either intellectually or emotionally with his situation. In the months before he was diagnosed, he had considerably more difficulty than most of those I interviewed in acknowledging that he might be infected with HIV. Although he had lost significant weight, experienced substantial pain, and seen his physical condition deteriorate, he had put off seeing a doctor as long as he could. As he explains, "I didn't want to find out I had AIDS. Even though I kind of figured I did, I didn't want to know. I wanted to live a normal life for as long as I could." Avoiding diagnosis and thus avoiding knowledge that was likely to be unpleasant had helped Kevin maintain his emotional health, despite his growing lack of control over his physical condition.

As Kevin's example demonstrates, those who downplay the importance of their symptoms, for whatever reason, may defer seeing a physician for some time. Of those who went for HIV testing only after they developed symptoms, almost every one did not seek medical care until they were sick enough to be diagnosed as having AIDS or ARC, rather than simply as HIV-infected. As the disease progresses, however, individuals eventually find that their health deteriorates to the point where they can no longer maintain their everyday living patterns and thus can no longer maintain the fiction that nothing is wrong. As their former ideas about the meaning of their symptoms crumble, persons with HIV disease face an intolerably ambiguous situation. Once they reach this point, the incentive grows to seek diagnosis and treatment.

Because the test for HIV was developed for use by blood banks, many public health workers worried when the test first appeared that gay men might donate blood so that they could get tested for HIV. As a result, the federal government funds at least one public blood-testing facility in every state so that gay men can learn whether they are infected without donating blood. Individuals who recognize that they might have HIV disease and go to one of these facilities soon have an explanation for their illness. Those who go to private physicians, however, may find it considerably more difficult to obtain a diagnosis. Many physicians simply lack the knowledge needed to diagnose HIV disease.[11] Others may not consider such diagnoses unless they know that their clients are at risk, even if their clients' symptoms fit the classic patterns for HIV disease. Yet some clients do not realize that they are at risk and others will not tell their physicians that they are at risk for fear of the stigma attendant on drug use or homosexual activity. These problems are probably most acute for those who live in areas where HIV disease is still relatively rare and still not very salient for doctors.

For all these reasons, then, persons with HIV disease may not receive accurate diagnoses until several months after they seek care. In the interim, and at least initially, some individuals accept or even welcome the alternative diagnoses that their physicians propose. When symptoms continue, however, they find themselves in what Stewart and Sullivan have described (with regard to multiple sclerosis) as "an ambiguous and uncertain limbo," in which they suffer anxieties about the meaning of their symptoms and cannot function normally, but in which those around them may neither believe that they are sick nor relieve them of any responsibilities.[12] Consequently, they cannot indefinitely sustain their own belief in these diagnoses.

To cope with this situation, some individuals will go from doctor to doctor to obtain a more believable diagnosis. Others research their symptoms, diagnose themselves, and then press their physicians to test for HIV. Even then, they may have difficulty obtaining a diagnosis. Several persons I interviewed complained that their physicians neither tested them for nor diagnosed them with HIV disease, even though they had classic symptoms (such as night sweats, persistent diarrhea, and weight loss), stated that they were gay, and requested that their blood be tested for HIV. Caleb, a forty-five-year-old mechanic, describes how his physician refused his several requests for testing, even though the physician knew he was gay and that something was wrong with his immune system. He says, "I was concerned. The symptoms were there, and I was not getting any better, not feeling any better, still getting weaker and weaker, losing more weight, and I kept mentioning all these things, and I said 'Look, I've been reading more articles about AIDS.' And he said, 'Oh, people are just panic-stricken. You don't have AIDS. I'm not doing a test on you.' " Stories such as this suggest that even when physicians have the necessary information, they may consciously or unconsciously avoid diagnosing HIV disease.

Diagnosis with HIV Disease

The experience of receiving one's diagnosis and the immediate aftermath of this experience vary widely from individual to individual. One critical factor is the doctor's familiarity with HIV disease. Those who suspect that they have HIV disease and seek diagnosis either at HIV testing facilities or from doctors who specialize in this illness usually receive sympathetic, detailed, and accurate information about their condition and prognosis. So do those who do not suspect that they have HIV disease but whose primary practitioners specialize in gay populations and therefore have become educated about this illness. The rest are not always so lucky. Unlike doctors in places like California or New York, most doctors in other parts of the country, such as Arizona, have little experience with

HIV disease. Consequently, although some doctors prove both sympathetic and knowledgeable, others make their ignorance and prejudice immediately known. They can do so by adopting unnecessary precautions against contagion such as donning gowns and masks, informing people who are infected with HIV but have yet to develop any opportunistic infections that they will die within a few months, speaking rudely or abruptly, and warning persons with HIV disease that they can infect their families if they hug them, cook their meals, or wash their clothes. Such stories were told to me by people diagnosed as recently as 1989.

The treatment Linda, Calvin, and Carrie received at diagnosis was considerably less humane than that received by the other people I interviewed, for these three had the misfortune to learn of their diagnosis while in "total institutions"—prison, a psychiatric hospital, and the military, respectively.[13] When prison authorities learned in 1986 that Linda had HIV disease, they transferred her from the minimum-security facility where she held a job outside the walls to isolation at a maximum-security prison. There she was served all her meals in her cell on Styrofoam plates and was segregated from other prisoners twenty-four hours a day. Similarly, that same year, when Calvin and his doctors at the county hospital psychiatric ward where he was receiving treatment following a suicide attempt learned that he had HIV disease, he was abruptly transferred to a maximum-security ward at the state mental hospital. According to Calvin:

> I was treated worse than a caged leopard. I was put in solitary confinement. I wasn't allowed to use the same bathroom as anybody else. I wasn't allowed to eat with the regular patients. All of my food came in disposable Styrofoam containers and they'd write on the container, "Calvin ———, isolation, AIDS." And the staff were very abusive, [telling me] "Stay away from me. I don't want you near me. . . ." The first night . . . two of them threw their keys down and quit. They weren't about to work with a faggot with AIDS.

Three years later, in 1989, Carrie was tested for HIV by the military. When her superior officer learned that she was infected with HIV, he immediately and without explanation relieved her of her duties and cancelled her upcoming leave. A few days later, and still with no explanation, he sent her to a doctor who told her she was infected and should "prepare to die." The doctor also told her she had probably infected her children, "did not deserve" ever to have sexual contact again, and should consider herself a "murderer" if she did so.

The reactions of persons with HIV disease to their diagnosis vary as widely as their doctors' reactions. At least at first, some individuals, whether diagnosed simply as HIV-infected or as having AIDS, assume that they can "beat" their illness. They thus refuse to take seriously any dire predictions about their future. Others cope with their situation by intellectually accepting that they have HIV disease but emotionally denying that fact. For example, two months after his diagnosis, Chris's doctor sent him to the hospital to test a culture the doctor had grown from a fungal infection on Chris's foot. Chris reports, "I'm reading this paper that he sent me over with and halfway down the paper it says, 'Caution: patient has AIDS,' and I almost turned around and walked back to him because I thought I had the wrong paper." Although this sort of denial cannot last long, it is comforting in the short run.

Conversely, other persons with HIV disease immediately consider their diagnosis "a death sentence"—again, whether they are asymptomatic but infected or whether they have AIDS. Carol, for example, has yet to develop any health problems. Nevertheless, she considers her prospects bleak. She says:

> The most difficult part [of being infected with HIV] is knowing you have no control over it. I'm a person that likes to be in control of my situation of whatever comes along. [With HIV,] you have control to make it worse, but you have no control to make it better. It's not like a cold that you know you're going to get over in a week. Or whatever it is.

Gonorrhea that you go and get a penicillin shot for. You have no control. It's there. And it's going to get you.

Five of the individuals I interviewed, including Carol, had attempted suicide shortly after their diagnosis, and several others had contemplated it often; other studies have conservatively estimated the rate of suicide among persons with AIDS to be from twenty-one to thirty-six times higher than that of the general population.[14] Others whom I interviewed had expressed their self-destructive feelings immediately following diagnosis in other ways, such as punching a hole in their living room wall or going on three-week drinking binges.

One reason Carol had tried to kill herself, and one reason she was among the most depressed and guilt-ridden individuals I interviewed, was that she had learned simultaneously that she was infected with HIV and that she had infected her newborn son. For two years before her diagnosis, Carol had been trying to get her husband to agree to a divorce. Consequently, when she accidentally became pregnant, she had difficulty truly acknowledging that fact. As a result, although during an earlier pregnancy she had stopped using illegal drugs and had not even used aspirin, during this pregnancy she occasionally injected cocaine. She knew she could put her fetus at risk by doing so, but did not want to believe that she was really pregnant. Describing how she felt when she learned that her baby was infected, Carol says, "I was so devastated at first I didn't care. It made no difference if I was going to be dead in two weeks or twenty years. I was just floored. And so ashamed of myself that I had used drugs during my pregnancy and that I had done this to my child. I felt like I had put a gun to his head and was just waiting to pull the trigger." Carol's sense of guilt "never goes away" and has overwhelmed her abilities to cope emotionally with her illness.

Following diagnosis, then, persons with HIV disease may experience a gamut of emotions, including guilt, depression, and fear. They also face a gamut of responses from others, ranging from sympathy to hostility, as they begin learning how to live with this new moral, social, and biological status. In subsequent days (and as the next chapter discusses), they face a series of decisions regarding when and with whom they should hide or reveal their new status—to try, in Goffman's terms, to remain "discreditable" rather than "discredited."[15]

The first such decision must be made before they leave their doctors' offices, for federal law requires doctors to report to the government the names of all persons with AIDS and Arizona law requires doctors to report all persons who are infected with HIV. Although laws supposedly protect the confidentiality of these reports, many physicians and patients fear that the information will leak out. As a result (and as Chapter 8 describes in more detail), to protect persons with HIV disease from possible legal, social, and financial repercussions, some doctors will bend the rules to avoid reporting. Similarly, individuals and their physicians may decide not to report diagnoses to insurance companies for fear the companies will terminate coverage or inform the individuals' employers. To further reduce the risk of stigma, some persons with HIV disease will request insurance reimbursement only for treatments that will not trigger questions about the nature of their diagnosis. Thus, from the time of diagnosis, individuals have to begin developing ways of coping with potential or actual stigma.

After Diagnosis: Explaining Why HIV Disease Strikes

Diagnosis with HIV disease ends individuals' uncertainty about what is wrong with them. It raises new questions, however, about why this terrible thing happened. Only by answering these questions can individuals make their illness comprehensible.

The search for meaning is often a painful one, set as it is in the context of popular belief that HIV disease is punishment for sin. At least on the surface, the majority of the individuals I interviewed reject the idea that their illness is a divine judgment.

Instead, those who believe in God stress that God is the source of love and not of punishment. In addition, gay persons with HIV disease often argue that God would not have created gay people only to reject them as sinners. These individuals and others I interviewed emphasize that HIV disease results from the same biological forces that cause other illnesses. Consequently, they dismiss the idea that they or anyone else deserve this illness. As David, a thirty-nine-year-old floral designer, says, "Nobody deserves it. I have friends that say 'well, hey, if we weren't gay, we wouldn't get this disease.' That's bullshit. I mean, I don't want to hear that from anybody. Because no germ has mercy on anybody, no matter who they are—gay, straight, babies, adults." Persons with HIV disease who agree with this philosophy may also bolster their argument by stressing that this illness originated with heterosexuals in Africa and thus could not be a punishment for homosexuality. They assert that it was simply bad luck that the first Americans infected with HIV were gay men or drug users.

These alternative explanations for their illnesses allow individuals to reject their rejecters as prejudiced or ignorant. Describing the Reverend Jerry Falwell's pronouncement that HIV disease is God's punishment for sin, Chris adds, "Somebody like that really ought to be put away. He's doing so much damage. It's pathetic and he doesn't know what he's talking about and that's real sad."

Yet in the same way that members of other oppressed groups sometimes feel they deserve their oppression, other statements by some of these same individuals suggest that at a less conscious level they do feel they are to blame for their illnesses.[16] For example, twenty-four-year-old Marshall denies that he deserves HIV disease, yet nevertheless suggests that his illness might be God's way of punishing him for being gay or "for not being a good person." He adds, "I should have helped people more, or not have yelled at somebody, or been better to my dad even though we have never gotten along. . . . Maybe if I had tried to get along better with him, maybe this wouldn't be happening."

Others maintain that they do not deserve HIV disease, but use language that suggests considerable ambivalence. Several, for example, attribute their illness not to their "nonmonogamy" or "multiple sexual partners" but rather to their "promiscuity." Chris, for example, believes he got HIV disease "probably because I was a royal whore for about four years." Others mention their "stupidity" or "carelessness." Their use of such morally loaded terms suggests that they are not simply describing their behavior objectively but rather are condemning it on moral grounds. Thus it seems they believe emotionally, if not intellectually, that they deserve punishment, although perhaps less severe punishment than HIV disease.

Still others have no doubt that they deserve HIV disease because of either their "immorality" or their lack of forethought in engaging in high-risk behaviors. For example, although at the time Daryl had convinced himself that HIV disease did not exist in Phoenix, in retrospect he blames himself for not taking more precautions. When asked how he felt when he learned his diagnosis, he replied, "Angry, I guess, at myself for allowing it to happen when I knew better. I mean, it's like, you deserve it. You knew what was going on and yet you slipped and this is the consequence." He reported feeling "disappointed in myself for allowing it to happen. It is something I brought on myself because I knew the possible consequences of what was going to happen."

Others explicitly state that they deserve HIV disease as punishment for activities they consider immoral. In these cases, diagnosis seems to unleash preexisting guilt about sexual activity or, to a much lesser extent, drug use. Such guilt seems particularly prevalent among gay men from fundamentalist Christian or Mormon families. Of the nine such persons I interviewed, five expressed regret about being gay and six at least partially believe that they deserve HIV disease. The most extreme reaction came from Brian, a thirty-five-year-old fundamentalist Christian. He says, "I reaped what I sowed. I sowed sin, I reaped death. I believe, biblically, I received AIDS as a result of my sexual sin practices." Such extreme feelings of self-blame are uncommon among the women, apparently because they never experienced such great conflicts about the behaviors that put them at risk.

The argument that HIV disease is a divine punishment can appear in inverse fashion among those who consider themselves innocent victims of this illness. Debbie, a middle-class mother and wife infected through a blood transfusion, says, "AIDS is a punishment from God. I just feel like he's telling the gay population to knock it off. And if they continue to do so, and infect each other knowingly, then they deserve what they get." She compared her own situation to that of the "innocent babies" whom the Bible says God killed to induce Pharaoh to release the Jews from Egypt: "There's always your innocent victims. We pay the price, but we're the ones that people stand up and look and get attention for, the innocent people and the babies."

None of the individuals I interviewed in 1986 or 1987 used Louise Hay's theory, which claims that illness is caused by individuals' lack of self-love, to explain their own illness (although one did use Hay's tapes for relaxation and inspiration). Of the twelve persons I interviewed in 1989, however, three are familiar with these ideas. Debbie's sister enrolled her in a seminar by Hay and added her name to Hay's mailing list. Although Debbie so far has resisted the pressures to adopt these theories, Sally and Sarah have concluded that they developed HIV disease because of their emotional conflicts over their sexual desires. Sally is a former call girl who wants to enter a legitimate occupation but misses the money and excitement of her former life, whereas Sarah believes that she was highly active sexually because she received little affection from her parents as a child. Belief in Hay's theory is probably more common on the two coasts, where it has gained the widest publicity, than in Arizona. Because so many gay magazines and newspapers have promoted Hay's view, it is also probably more common among gay men than among others at risk for HIV disease. Such ideas will become more common in the future, as they continue to spread from the two coasts to the interior and from gays to mainstream society. The local Phoenix newsletter for persons with HIV disease, for example, seems to print an increasing number of articles on the topic with each passing year.

Not all persons with HIV disease, however, have found it necessary to attribute blame to themselves or others in an effort to explain their illness. Instead, and despite the price exacted by their illness, five of the thirty-seven men and women I interviewed define their illness in positive terms as a gift from God. Brent, a thirty-three-year-old computer operator and a staunch Catholic, considers his illness to be a divine gift rather than divine retribution. In the past, his disastrous choice of lovers had left him suicidal on several occasions. As a result, he regards his illness literally as an "answer to a prayer," because it provides the extra incentive he needs to avoid any further romantic entanglements. In slightly different fashion, Carrie, Grace, Sarah, and Jeremy have found benefits in their illness by adopting an altruistic perspective. Carrie, Grace, and Sarah are heterosexual women with firm religious convictions who have never injected illegal drugs. They believe that God has given them this illness to increase their compassion, sensitivity, and ability to work with those less fortunate than themselves and to enable them to champion the rights of all persons with HIV disease, including those who are far less likely to receive sympathy from the general public. Similarly, Jeremy, a twenty-six-year-old gay fundamentalist Christian, believes his illness has helped him pursue his lifelong goals of improving the position of gays and sharing his religious faith with others. As he explains:

> The only thing that I can actually think of, the only reason why I would get AIDS, . . . is the fact that I really feel that me getting AIDS has opened a lot of doors for me to share with people—either gay people who feel that God rejects them because they're gay, but even more so to the "Christian" community who refuse to accept homosexuals as being Christian. That's the only reason I can think of, is because I know I'm a Christian, and I can share this with certain people. I've got to share the things that have happened. Since I've got AIDS, I've

been able to share the fact that you can be a homosexual and still go to heaven with people up in [rural towns] and all over. Just unbelievable.

All four individuals are working to improve the position of persons with HIV disease, and all have spoken publicly about their situations. In addition, Carrie is planning on filing an antidiscrimination suit against her employer, the military.

Regardless of how an individual explains why he or she got HIV disease, simply having an explanation makes it easier to tolerate the illness. For this reason, those who believe that others deserve to contract this illness, but that they themselves do not, appear the most distressed. They rage at the unfairness of their situation. Jeanne, for example, feels that HIV disease is fitting punishment for gays, but not for drug users like herself, while Marshall says, "I get real angry. I don't know how to explain why I got it and somebody else didn't because I don't consider myself that I was that promiscuous. When I go out, I see other guys out in the bars and they're hopping around, two and three guys a night basically. And it's like why aren't they getting it? Why is it me?" Individuals who engage in such downward social comparison increase the anxiety caused by uncertainty about why this has happened to them, but decrease their feelings of stigma by labeling others more immoral or deviant than themselves.[17]

Having HIV disease is also particularly distressful for those who believe they could not have avoided contracting the illness. Those who believe they were born gay consider it unfair that their innate sexual orientation put them at risk for HIV disease, whereas those who had quit using drugs before becoming ill feel that they are being punished unfairly for past sins. Such persons must cope with both the physical trauma of illness and the emotional trauma of losing their faith that this is a just world. Calvin vividly describes what this feels like:

I often put myself in the situation of standing in a courtroom and trying to justify what I did and why I did it, but the judge and jury have decided, and the courtroom is empty and nobody is there but me. They've already sentenced me, and I'm standing there saying, "Hey, yoo hoo. Wait a minute. I've got something to say! Wait! You don't understand. There's a reason I did what I did!" And all you get is a hollowing echo, and there's nobody home, nobody listening. You just stand there with no one to turn to and you say, "So be it, I understand." And you go on with what's left.

Envisioning the Future

Diagnosis with HIV disease forces individuals to begin reconstructing their image of what their futures will be like. Because this illness can affect the body in so many ways, it is difficult to know what to expect. Some will become blind because of infection with cytomegalovirus, some will become disabled because of tuberculosis, and some will live for months or even years with only minimal health problems. Consequently, individuals face tremendous uncertainty about the nature of their remaining days.

Fear of death is minimal compared to fear of what one's life may become. In particular, individuals fear that they will be among the approximately 40 percent who suffer mild neurological impairment, the 10 percent who suffer true dementia, or the 10 percent who become disfigured by the lesions of Kaposi's sarcoma.[18] In addition, they especially fear esoteric illnesses whose effects they cannot predict. As Jeremy says, "I'm not [as] afraid of getting infections from people as I am from inanimate objects, like fruits and moldy tile. . . . I know what a cold is like. . . . [It's] something that I have experienced. I've never experienced a mold infection."

Persons with HIV disease have little control over whether they will develop such infections. To cope with this lack of control, some try to maintain unrealistic images of their futures by avoiding learning about their illness. Kevin, who had put off diagnosis as long as he could, also put off learning about HIV disease. He echoes the sentiments of several others when he explains that he has not joined a support group for persons with this illness because he does not "want to see what other people look like." Such feelings are especially common among persons at earlier stages of HIV disease and among those at later stages who, like Kevin, seem especially distraught over their situations. These individuals fear that gaining knowledge will lead to depression and therefore conclude that they can better cope with uncertainty about the future by maintaining ignorance.

Other individuals cope with uncertainty and lack of control by developing realistic predictions about their futures. To learn about the consequences and treatments of various infections (and to obtain emotional support), individuals may attend support groups offered by community organizations that deal with HIV disease. They can also research their illnesses on their own, and in some cases they develop extensive libraries on the subject. The knowledge that they gain allows them to feel that they can respond appropriately should some problem arise, and thus can exert some control over their situations.

This strategy, however, is really only available to those who live in major cities. In smaller cities and towns, libraries and bookstores are often too small to help, and support groups may not exist. In Arizona, only Tucson and Phoenix have support groups. Persons who live in other cities may not even know that these groups exist. Debbie, for example, who lives in an outlying city of about fifty thousand people, only learned of the community organizations that deal with HIV disease through our interview, even though she was diagnosed three years earlier and receives most of her care in a major Arizona treatment center for HIV disease. Moreover, if she had wanted to attend a group, she would have had to travel more than two hundred miles each way to do so.

Even if they live in major cities, heterosexuals with HIV disease may have trouble getting the information they need. The medical literature on HIV disease largely relies on studies conducted on gay men or, less commonly, men who use intravenous drugs. Given the highly variable course of HIV disease, that literature is not necessarily applicable to any women or to men who contract this illness in other ways. Similarly, support groups and community organizations for persons with HIV disease cannot answer all the questions heterosexuals have because they, too, rely primarily on the shared experiences of gay men for their knowledge. In addition, even if support groups can provide useful information, heterosexuals may not attend because they consider the groups to be essentially gay social events, feel angry at gay men who they believe caused the epidemic, or, like many Americans, are uncomfortable interacting with gay people. To date, all attempts in Arizona to start a support group solely for women have failed. Attempts to start a group for drug users have been only partially successful, with the single resulting group meeting intermittently.

Questions about the future are difficult to answer for those who initially receive diagnoses of ARC or chronic HIV infection rather than AIDS, and even more difficult for those who learn while still asymptomatic that they are infected with HIV. Faced with conflicting estimates of when and whether they will develop AIDS, such persons experience enormous stress. Interviewed after her first negative ELISA test, Grace, the woman whose HIV status remains undetermined, said, "I'm not excited. I'm not relieved. I'm puzzled. And I'm not going to accept it at face value. . . . I don't feel that just this one negative ELISA is enough to make me go out and open a bottle of champagne and celebrate." Instead, she has concluded that it is emotionally safer to assume that she is infected with HIV than to assume that she is not and risk having her hopes dashed. She stated that she would rather know that she was positive than continue not knowing, "Because for me, personally, in all areas of my life, not knowing is harder for me. I can take the truth and deal with it. Not knowing, I have a harder time dealing with it." Brent echoes her feeling in describing how his emotional state changed when his diagnosis changed from ARC (at the time of the first interview) to AIDS (at the time of the six-month follow-up interview). He says, "The worst feeling was when I was ARC, waiting for a bomb to explode. Not knowing when or if ever it would do it. There was always that tentative in my life that it may or may not. Beware! Now that the diagnosis has come in, it's like 'Okay. I can relax now. The worst is over.' " As these quotes suggest, for many individuals, even the most devastating knowledge is preferable to living with uncertainty.

Conclusions

The process of becoming a person with HIV disease centers around coming to terms with uncertainty. Although uncertainty is a central concern for all seriously ill persons, it seems to have an especially great impact on those who have HIV disease. First, persons with this illness are more likely than most ill persons to know prior to diagnosis that they are at risk. As a result, they experience difficulties other ill persons do not, for uncertainty and anxiety often sap their emotional energy and physical resources months or even years before they become ill. Second, persons with HIV disease are more likely to feel guilt about the behaviors that led to their illness and, consequently, to believe that they deserve their illness. Moreover, these individuals are far more likely to find that their friends, families, and the general public also believe that they caused and deserve their illness. As a result, these others often reinforce the guilt that persons with HIV disease feel. Third, persons with HIV disease are more likely to face difficulties in obtaining an accurate diagnosis. Like other illnesses, HIV disease can be difficult to diagnose because it is rare and causes multiple symptoms. These problems are exacerbated when physicians deliberately (if unconsciously) avoid questions or actions that would lead to diagnosis. Fourth, persons with HIV disease face greater uncertainty than other ill persons in predicting how their illness will affect their lives, for HIV disease causes more extensive and less predictable physical and mental damage than most other illnesses. Finally, because HIV disease is such a new disease, infected individuals are more likely than other ill persons to lack answers to their questions about treatment and prognosis. Moreover, because physicians' understanding of HIV disease is rapidly developing and constantly changing, persons who have this illness often are reluctant to trust the answers they do receive.

Uncertainty seems particularly troubling for persons with HIV disease who are not gay men. These individuals face additional problems in obtaining diagnoses because they may not know they are at risk. Some women, for example, do not know that their male partners are bisexual. Other men and women believe that only gays are at risk. Moreover, their physicians may be less alert for and knowledgeable about HIV disease than the physicians of gay men, who in many instances specialize in gay health care. Following diagnosis with HIV disease, individuals who are not gay, and especially women, also experience more difficulty in predicting their futures because most studies have only investigated how HIV disease affects gay men. In addition, they are far less likely to have networks of fellow sufferers to turn to for advice and information. Some live on the margins of society and lack either access to or knowledge of community resources. Others are either unwilling because of their own homophobia to accept help from groups dominated by gay men or are unable to get help because their problems are too different from those of gay men. Finally, heterosexuals with HIV disease may suffer greater uncertainty about whether they might transmit HIV to others. Although most gay men with HIV disease also worry about infecting sexual partners, they function in social circles where everyone is presumed to be at risk. Consequently, their fear of infecting others generally does not have the same overwhelming quality as that experienced by heterosexuals who believe that they are the sole potential source of infection for their loved ones.

Despite all the difficulties persons with HIV disease face because of uncertainty, however, they are not helpless against it. Rather, they can find ways to reduce or, if necessary, to live with uncertainty. These data highlight the role that control plays in making uncertainty tolerable. Persons with HIV disease cope with uncertainty by developing normative frameworks that make their situations comprehensible. Even when inaccurate, these frameworks help individuals choose (albeit from among limited options) how they will live their lives. They therefore help persons with HIV disease feel at least minimally in control. In the final analysis, it is this sense of control that enables these individuals to live with uncertainty.

CHAPTER 5

HIV Disease
and the Body

At the time they learn that they are infected with HIV, some people still feel healthy and strong, as do some who already have recovered from their first opportunistic infections. In future years, treatments may be developed that will keep persons infected with HIV from developing AIDS, and keep persons with AIDS from dying. Indeed, some observers already refer to HIV disease as a manageable illness. At present, however, it is reasonable for persons with HIV disease to expect that their immune systems will gradually weaken, leading to increasing disability and eventual death. This chapter describes the struggles of persons with HIV disease to find good health care providers, their attempts to retain control over their bodies for as long as possible, and how their lives and self-concepts change once they begin losing that control.

Finding Health Care Providers

Both to keep themselves as healthy as possible and to deal with health problems as they arise, persons with HIV disease must depend on health care providers. An early task individuals face following diagnosis, therefore, is finding a skilled and caring primary practitioner.

This is not necessarily easy, especially for those who live far from the original centers of the epidemic. Although Link and his colleagues found that 75 percent of interns and residents at four New York City hospitals where HIV disease is common would willingly continue to treat persons with HIV disease, their sample is unusual, because such hospitals undoubtedly attract persons willing to do so.[1] Other studies have found that up to 76 percent of doctors would prefer not to treat persons with HIV disease because they either fear infection or believe such persons do not deserve their services.[2]

Finding a doctor is easiest for individuals (usually gay men) who know of other persons with HIV disease or community organizations that can provide recommendations. Finding a doctor is most difficult for those who are unfamiliar with such networks and who, additionally, live outside of major cities. Debbie, for example, diagnosed three years ago, still has not found a primary practitioner in her small city who will treat a person with HIV disease. Instead, for primary care, she relies on her ear, nose, and throat doctor, who volunteered to accept this responsibility because she has been his patient for many years.

Eventually, through trial and error, most do find primary practitioners who they believe provide good and nonjudgmental care. They still can encounter problems, however, whenever they need to see a specialist, go to a hospital, or find a nursing home or after-care facility. In Arizona, as in many other states, relatively few specialists, only a handful of ambulance services, and no nursing home or after-care facility will care for persons with HIV disease. (However, one of the local community organizations that deals with HIV disease recently received a federal grant to open a nursing home.)

In most situations, the responsibility for finding a specialist lies with the individual's primary practitioner rather than with the individual. Nevertheless, this search still takes an emotional toll, for persons with HIV disease know that many doctors do not want to work with them and fear that they may receive substandard care from doctors who will treat them only grudgingly.

The one situation in which individuals retain primary responsibility is finding a dentist. This is not a minor issue, for dental complications commonly accompany HIV disease and can seriously limit individuals' quality of life. Because dental work is a form of surgery, dentists fear that they will be infected by splashed blood. Consequently, dentists are one of the groups least willing to provide care to persons with HIV disease. In Arizona, only a handful of dentists will do so. Moreover, these few dentists try to keep word of their availability from spreading, because they fear that they will attract too many such patients and will consequently scare away other patients. This is not an unreasonable fear; Gerbert and her colleagues found that 25 percent of individuals surveyed in a nationwide random sample would change doctors if they learned that their doctor treated persons with HIV disease.[3] As a result, persons with HIV disease find it enormously difficult to find a sympathetic dentist. Consequently, many defer dental care longer than is wise.

Persons with HIV disease have even fewer options when it comes to emergency care. In such circumstances, they usually cannot choose their ambulance service, hospital, or doctor. In Arizona and much of the country still, as in New York or California several years ago, ambulance services may refuse to pick up patients known to be infected with HIV. In other cases, they will pick up patients but will provide a lower quality of care.

The same holds true for hospital staff. No hospital can refuse to accept persons with HIV disease simply on the basis of their diagnosis (although they can use patients' economic status as an excuse for refusing care). The quality of care hospital staff provide to such persons can vary tremendously, however. Although some staff provide excellent care to all regardless of diagnosis, others refuse care or provide care only grudgingly. Several individuals, both in the earliest and the most recent interviews, mentioned social workers who refused to enter their hospital rooms and hospital staff who refused to provide care or disappeared without warning once their diagnoses became known. Jeremy, for example, first realized that he had HIV disease when his original hospital staff team disappeared and was replaced by a new team, all of whom appeared to be gay. Susan, a twenty-seven-year-old bartender and former drug user, as well as a wife and mother of two, describes a similar incident:

> This lady came in to take my blood and she's shaking. My husband's sitting on the end of the bed. She has these gloves on. That doesn't bother me, that's great. That's for protection. She's shaking. I said, "Lady do you want me to do that? If you're that nervous, please go get somebody else that can handle this, because I don't want you sticking nothing in my arm like that." "Okay, I will," she said. My IV came out of my arm, and it's pumping blood out. I rang for the nurse, and blood's everywhere. I mean everywhere. And, it was so funny. The nurse comes in and says, "Oh my God!" She puts on the gloves and everything. Do you know that blood stayed there until the day I left? Nobody cleaned my room. *I* cleaned it.

As bad as the care Susan received was, it is still better than the care individuals may receive if they live in smaller cities where hospital staff have even less knowledge about HIV disease. For this reason, Debbie's doctor has warned her that, whenever possible, she should seek hospital and specialist care at a larger city more than two hundred miles away rather than in her own city.

A major dilemma persons with HIV disease face whenever they must seek care from anyone other than their regular provider is deciding whether to disclose their diagnosis. If they do, they risk either rejection or receiving poor-quality care. If they do not, they risk receiving unsatisfactory care from workers who do not understand the nature of their health problems. In addition, they must bear the emotional burden of knowing that they can expose these workers to HIV. Grace describes the mental turmoil she went through when she needed medical assistance following a camping accident:

> I had an accident this weekend where there was a lot of blood. I was taken to the emergency room at [the nearest small city] and morally, ethically, whatever, could not determine what to do. There was part of me that wanted to say, "Hey gang, I'm HIV-positive, you need to be taking precautions." But the other part of me said, "Yeah, but then will you get any kind of good care?" So instead, I utilized the fact of where I worked [at a community organization that deals with HIV disease] and talked about universal precautions and were they going to use universal precautions? . . . Those are things you would never think about. Six months ago it would [have gotten] not a second's thought. Instead it was the only thing on my mind from the time of the accident until I was out of the hospital. . . . I spent the whole time wondering what do I owe these people that are taking care of me and what do I owe myself?

In similar circumstances, others have decided that they must inform health care providers of their illness, regardless of any costs to themselves. Still others believe that, because so many patients do not know that they are infected with HIV, all health care workers should know enough to use standard precautions against infection with all patients. They therefore argue that workers who do not use standard precautions have only themselves to blame if they get infected, and feel no obligation to disclose their diagnosis.

This issue has caused frequent arguments between Debbie and her husband. Because of her fears of infecting others, Debbie bought a "medic alert" bracelet etched with her diagnosis. Her husband, fearing that paramedics might refuse to care for her if they saw it, threw it out. She reports that he told her, "They can find out after the fact. And if they weren't smart enough to put their gloves on and their face masks on, they deserve whatever they get. But I'm not going to have you dying because they're afraid of you."

Because of the dearth of physicians outside of certain major coastal cities willing to treat persons with HIV disease, and because of financial constraints that force such persons to accept whatever doctors the indigent health care system provides, persons with HIV disease have few choices about what doctors they see. As a result, they may have to accept care from doctors who, although technically competent, do not meet their needs in other ways.

Most importantly, persons with HIV disease desire doctors who will give them the information they need to make informed choices from among their options, rather than doctors who will treat them like children who cannot make such decisions for themselves. In this respect, persons with HIV disease are no different from any patients who seek active roles in their health care. Some persons with HIV disease do find doctors, particularly those trained as primary practitioners, who like sharing their decision-making authority with patients. Others, especially those who must rely on specialists (and including those infectious disease specialists who become primary practitioners for persons with HIV disease), find that their doctors are uncomfortable with such an untraditional doctor-patient relationship. Hugh, for example, is a twenty-nine-year-old blue-collar worker with ARC. He is constantly frustrated with the way his doctor resists sharing information with him, telling him "everything is going to be fine" and "don't worry about it, I'm here." Hugh has found this very frustrating. However, because so few doctors are willing to treat persons with HIV disease, he feels he has no choice.

In addition, persons with HIV disease seek doctors who will acknowledge the emotional as well as the physical impact of illness, help them cope with their feelings, and deal with them as persons rather than as bodies and organs. Again, primary practitioners, especially if they are gay and treat many persons with HIV disease, are most likely to do this. Brent's doctor has one of the largest case loads of persons with HIV disease in the state. Brent says, "[My doctor] treats me as a real human being. He gives me a hug every time I come in and he's not afraid to touch me. [He] makes me feel good, . . . like a human being, not like a diseased person." Other persons with HIV disease, however, are not so lucky, and must bear these emotional burdens without assistance from the one group of persons that knows the most about their illness.

Seeking Treatments and Cures

Regardless of where or from whom individuals receive their medical care, they must decide what strategies will preserve their health the longest. This is true both for those who assume that diagnosis with HIV disease is a death sentence and for those who assume from the start, or conclude once the initial shock is over, that they can "beat" their illness.

The methods individuals adopt to protect their health vary widely. Some rely primarily on prayer; others use prayer to supplement other methods. In addition, they strive to eat more balanced meals, take vitamins, get regular exercise, reduce stress in their lives, develop a positive attitude, and limit their use of caffeine, tobacco, and illegal drugs. They try to limit their exposure to germs by, for example, avoiding animals and swimming pools and scanning public buses for passengers who looked unhealthy before choosing a seat. And they may seek any potential treatments, including experimental, illegal, or toxic ones, that might increase their chances for survival.

All these tactics have associated costs. Changing one's lifestyle is never easy, and can result in feelings of loss as one gives up pleasures in exchange for the possibility of a longer life. Carol, for example, has yet to develop any health problems as a result of HIV. To preserve her health, she has been told to stop drinking, taking drugs, lying in the sun, and eating various pleasurable foods. She describes the difficulties this advice presents:

You really don't appreciate things until you have to give them up. Like . . . there's certain things that they say don't eat. You know, don't eat yeast, and don't eat white bread because of the flour and processed sugar. And one of the first things they told me was that caffeine and carbonation are bad for the AIDS virus. I hardly ever drink soda. I wanted a soda so bad, I couldn't stand it. And I'm not a sweet eater, and I must have went through ten cans of Almond Roca candy. I don't eat candy. I couldn't get enough. . . . It's kind of like getting in a motorcycle accident and being paralyzed. You wouldn't realize how much walking meant until you lose it.

Seeking medical treatments presents another set of difficulties and trade-offs. Although standard treatments exist for many opportunistic infections, and the main drug used against HIV itself, zidovudine (formerly called azidothymidine or AZT), is no longer classified as experimental, persons with HIV disease still must rely heavily on experimental drugs if they are to stay relatively healthy.

By definition, one can never know the potential hazards of experimental treatments. Any drug toxic enough to stop HIV, however, is likely to be toxic to individuals' bodies as well. For example, the standard treatment for HIV disease is now zidovudine. Preliminary research reports from the manufacturer suggest that at low dosages, zidovudine is both effective and safe. At the dosages in which it was originally administered, however, zidovudine often resulted in overwhelming nausea, headaches, and loss of red and white blood cells. The nausea could be so severe that individuals felt incapable of eating. The headaches could make individuals feel that life itself was not worthwhile. And the loss of blood cells could be life-threatening. Thus, using an experimental drug—even one that proves useful in the long run—always involves risks and is never a simple decision.

Despite these hazards, when faced with the prospects of an early death, persons with HIV disease may go to extraordinary lengths to obtain any promising treatments. Zidovudine provides a good example of what this can entail. At the time of the first interviews, in 1986 and 1987, individuals could get zidovudine legally only if they were among the few chosen to participate in pharmaceutical experiments. The rest had to rely on various subterfuges to obtain it. Some convinced their physicians to diagnose them inaccurately so they would meet the experimenters' criteria. Some received zidovudine from physicians who continued collecting pills from drug researchers for patients who had died. Others obtained unused pills from friends who were research subjects. These friends gave away pills that they had been instructed by the experimenters to destroy, either because they had forgotten to take their pills on schedule or because they had skipped them to avoid side effects that they found intolerable. Friends could also obtain an extra set of pills to give away by registering as research subjects under two names with two physicians.

As a result of pressure from persons with HIV disease to make new drugs more rapidly available, the federal government recently loosened its restrictions on experimental drugs for HIV disease. As a result, experimental drugs now can be released on the market after only brief, preliminary tests. This does not, however, guarantee individuals the drugs they desire. Zidovudine, for example, is now available by prescription, but costs about $8,000 per year (down from an original price of $12,000).[4] These prices make it effectively unavailable to many men and women. Even those who have health insurance often find that their insurance does not cover drugs, especially those classified as experimental. Insurance plans that do pay for drugs typically reimburse patients for only 80 percent of the cost. The remaining 20 percent (which would come to about $1,600 yearly for zidovudine alone) is beyond the means of many persons with HIV disease. As a result, individuals can only obtain desired drugs if they are willing and able to accumulate enormous debts or if their illness has already bankrupted them and they live in a state that provides these drugs through Medicaid or its equivalent. Newer experimental drugs, meanwhile, continue to be available only to persons with HIV disease who qualify for and have access to research programs. Because the federal government has located almost all centers for testing experimental drugs for HIV disease on the two coasts, individuals in other parts of the country typically have no legal means of obtaining such drugs.[5] As a result, the underground market continues to thrive for other new drugs, which persons with HIV disease and their friends either manufacture or import from countries where they are legally available; one study found that 28 percent of AIDS patients in San Francisco are taking illegal medications, often without their doctors' knowledge.[6]

In addition to changing their lifestyles and seeking medical treatments, individuals can also try to increase their chances for survival by adopting a positive attitude. As Clint, a thirty-one-year-old entrepreneur diagnosed with AIDS, explains, "The main killer with having AIDS is that mental psyche, because your mind controls your body. . . . There are so many people that can't get past that 'I'm sick and going to die.' And therefore, they don't even start—they die." He and others like him strive to maintain their health by refusing to believe that they will die and by acting on that belief. Similarly, Tom, a thirty-eight-year-old administrator diagnosed with ARC, says that he has not written a will because of "that whole will-to-live bit. Once I get that done, that means one less thing I have to do. As long as I don't have it done, it seems like, well, I can't die yet." Instead of planning for their deaths, therefore, persons with HIV disease at whatever stage may consciously plan for their lives—buying cars on two-year loans, registering for concert series, or the like.

To encourage a positive attitude, persons with HIV disease may seek any course of action that will help them believe that they can control their fate and thus help them maintain their hope of survival. Thus Tom stresses the importance of "being active about this disease, whether it involves drinking a certain kind of tea or standing on your head twice a day or doing something, something that gives the patient a feeling of control over his own life that if you do these things, this might help you a little bit." As he explains, "It's a sense of being in control, of being actively involved in your own health, which in itself produces health."

Extending this philosophy, some persons with HIV disease consciously work to improve their mental attitudes through visualization and affirmation exercises. For this reason, Sally, who has ARC, has not only given up smoking, drinking, fatty foods, and late nights out dancing, but also listens regularly to Louise Hay's tapes of affirmations. In addition, during an extended period in which she could not walk, she used visualization exercises. She explains, "I had put up photographs of me in high heels. It sounds like really funny, but I was more upset that I couldn't go dancing in high heels than not being able to walk. Because I love my high heels and I love dancing. So I put up the photos, and I tried to visualize myself dancing." Although she lacks the necessary faith to get retested for HIV, she believes that these affirmations and visualizations have cured her.

HIV Disease and the Body

In the short run, adopting a healthier lifestyle, seeking treatments, and maintaining a positive attitude can help individuals remain relatively healthy and feel in control despite uncertainty about their futures. At present, however, and given the state of medical knowledge, persons with HIV disease can expect eventually to experience considerable physical disability. Fevers, rashes, nausea, diarrhea, exhaustion, pain, and difficulty breathing are common. Describing his "bad" days, Brian says, "All I can do is lay down and breathe and sometimes I feel like that's going to be quite a chore." On his "good" days, he can get up, but "just walking from there to here [across the room] would be real rough."

The loss of physical abilities is particularly apparent and important to individuals who previously had prided themselves on those abilities. For example, in the past, Hugh would go out and dance all night. He says, "The longest I've ever done it was sixteen hours straight of nonstop dancing. And I used to get up in four hours after that and feel great. . . . I was a very healthy, strong male. And to see that I can't even walk up to the blasted mailbox and back without huffing and puffing and feeling like I just ran the marathon really bothers me."

These bodily changes threaten individuals' self-concepts by presenting them with unequivocal evidence that their former ideas of who they are no longer are accurate. Moreover, persons with HIV disease find it especially difficult to accept the changes in their physical abilities because those changes are so unpredictable. Even those individuals who are convinced that in the long run HIV disease will drain their strength and kill them soon find that the course of the illness over the short run is highly idiosyncratic. Persons with HIV disease can never know when a new infection will further sap their energy. Nor can they know when or if an infection will end or how long a remission will last. As a result, they can never know from one day to the next how sick they will be. Daryl, who has AIDS, explains, "Probably the hardest thing is not knowing when you're well what's going to happen tomorrow. Because when you're well all you're thinking about is, 'What am I going to get? What's the next infection I'm going to have to put up with?' Of course, when you're sick it's like, 'Well, I hope they can make me well. I wonder if they can or not?' "

Even those whose health problems are still relatively minor can lose the sense that they control their bodies. Debbie, for example, has yet to suffer a serious opportunistic infection. Nevertheless, she describes the sense of frustration her problematic health has caused:

I want to continue being the person that lives in my brain. The body won't follow along. The energy is not there. I can't be going from the time I get up 'til the time I go to bed. I can't be tap dancing at ten o'clock at night. And I hate that. I hate it that I can't. . . . I'm still me in my head but my body is HIV-infected and that's hard that I can't [do those things]. Because you think it's mind over matter. But it's not. It's gotten to the point now that it's matter over mind.

As the illness progresses, individuals also lose control over their appearance, further threatening their self-concepts. In the later stages of the illness, individuals often become emaciated, obviously weak, or marked by rashes or cancer lesions. Linda, for example, who has ARC, describes herself half-humorously as looking "like a poster child for feed the starving children." They therefore become unable to maintain the "front," or physical image that they need to sustain their previous and desired self-images.[7] These damaged fronts create feelings of great loss, especially among persons who had prided themselves previously on their looks. Hugh explains:

> People say, "You really don't look that much different. You look thinner, but you don't really look that much different." And I'd say, "Yeah, but you're not me. You don't know what it's like to lose that much all at once. You don't know what it's like to lose four inches across the chest, and knowing that it was all muscle, and two inches on the arm, and knowing that it was all muscle."

In addition to creating a sense of loss, changes in appearance also force persons with HIV disease to recognize that their health has deteriorated. Calvin, who has AIDS, seemed in physical pain throughout our interview. He says, "When I look in the mirror and I see the change, and the sinking of the face, the color that I've lost, when I can actually see and meet face-to-face the physical changes, then . . . you realize [your situation]. The first time that I looked at myself in the mirror and saw the change was the first acceptance I had that I was at the beginning of the end."

Because of the erratic course of HIV disease, infected individuals can neither take their health for granted nor count on being ill. As a result, they lose the sense of control over their lives. This becomes an especially critical issue with regard to making long-range plans. Because persons with HIV disease can become incapacitated without warning, they expose themselves to possible disappointment whenever they make such plans. For example, Sally, a thirty-five-year-old college dropout, is considering taking a nine-month technical training course. She worries that the stress of school may harm her health and that her poor health may keep her from completing her schoolwork. As a result, she feels she is "living in limbo. Because how are you supposed to plan a future if you don't know if you have a future?" Even making short-range plans can become a source of stress and anxiety for the more sickly individuals. For example, Chris, who has AIDS, fears going "for a little trip tomorrow even though I am capable of doing that, but I may have diarrhea, and who wants to be driving down the highway with shit in your pants?"

These problems lead some of the sicker individuals to protect themselves against disappointment by never making plans.[8] By thus acknowledging their lack of control over their physical health, they hope to assert control over their emotional health. For example, Calvin says, "AIDS has become my life. I live for AIDS. I don't live for me anymore, I live for AIDS. I'm at its beck and call, and I'll do what it tells me when it tells me." Calvin now spends most of his days watching television in his trailer.

Although avoiding plans protects persons with HIV disease against disappointment, it increases their frustration. As Chris explains, "I may have a day where I feel great, where I have plenty of energy and everything is fine, and then you have nothing going, you're just sitting there in the house rotting. So that is really frustrating." Consequently, individuals must walk a tightrope—making the plans needed to lead a meaningful life without inviting disappointment when those plans collapse. For this reason, several compare themselves to recovering alcoholics, who must learn to live "one day at a time."

The physical deterioration caused by HIV disease directly affects how individuals view their sexuality and how their sexuality is viewed by others. This is a critical and devastating impact of having this illness, for sexuality is a basic part of everyone's self-concept. It is especially salient for gay men, for it both sets them apart from most people and ties them to other gays. Moreover, sexual activity forms a major part of many gay men's lives. In one large survey of gay men in San Francisco conducted early in the epidemic of HIV disease, respondents reported an average of 3.2 different sexual partners per month, and in a recent survey conducted in the Phoenix, Arizona area, respondents reported an average of 1.1 partners per month.[9]

The loss of physical strength experienced by persons with HIV disease makes it difficult for them to perform sexually. At the same time, if they either had no partner before their diagnosis or were abandoned by their partner following diagnosis, their loss of attractiveness makes it difficult to find new sexual partners. Even if their partners do not abandon them, the partners may curtail sexual contact out of fear of infection. In addition, because most persons with HIV disease contracted their illness through sexual activity and all can spread it sexually, many lose their sexual desire. Douglas, a thirty-four-year-old financial planner, does not consider homosexuality immoral but now finds it physically repulsive. As he explains, "Homosexual sex to me now is just something that is vile. It caused me to have a horrible disease. . . . The desire for it is gone, so what is left basically is the association with disease and death and sickness. . . . I just can't conceive of having sex right now. It is just something that I don't want. It's nauseous to me."

Other persons with HIV disease remain interested in sex, but, because they must abandon or drastically alter long-established sexual habits to protect others from infection, conclude that sex is no longer worthwhile. Several men, for example, compare having sex while wearing condoms to "taking a shower with a raincoat on." They therefore have chosen abstinence. Other men and women have ceased sexual activity because they feel that all sexual activities, no matter how careful, carry the risk of infecting one's partner. They therefore equate having sex with "playing Russian roulette with someone else's life" or even "committing murder." Still others are unwilling to have sex because, based on what their doctors have told them, they fear that they can become reinfected with the virus and become more ill if they do so. For a variety of reasons, therefore, persons with HIV disease may conclude that celibacy is their best option. Even when this choice is freely made, however, the loss of physical and emotional intimacy can cause significant emotional distress.

Whenever illness devastates the body, it is natural for individuals to turn to their intellect as an alternative source of satisfaction and self-esteem. As Cheri Register documents in her research on chronic illness, many ill persons distance themselves emotionally from their bodies, comforting themselves with the thought that as long as their minds remain intact, their true selves have not changed.[10] The most terrifying aspect of HIV disease, therefore, is its ability to ravage mind as well as body.

Both HIV itself and the consequent opportunistic infections can cause neurological impairment. Most medical authorities estimate that about half of persons infected with HIV eventually suffer some mental impairment, although some preliminary findings suggest that the new antiviral drugs may make this less common.[11] About 10 percent experience true dementia, whereas the rest experience headaches, forgetfulness, inability to concentrate, blindness, or a general slowing in thinking.

The possibility of mental impairment is a great source of stress to persons with HIV disease. Moreover, because the decline in mental abilities can develop gradually, individuals may be aware of the changes as they occur. This awareness itself causes suffering. Clint, for example, says, "I don't seem to be able to read. And I like to and I want to read, but it seems to run together. And at various times I just can't seem to concentrate. That bothers me because I wanted to keep my brain skills going. I don't feel as intelligent as I felt. I really don't. It seems like I can't reach out and grasp what I used to reach out and grasp mentally." As this quote suggests, neurological problems can make it difficult or impossible for individuals to sustain successful performances and thus can significantly damage their self-concepts.

As both mind and body deteriorate, persons with HIV disease must seek help from others with routine housekeeping chores. By the end of their lives, as well as during periods of acute illness, they need help with feeding, clothing, washing themselves, and eliminating bodily wastes. Although Sally was healthy enough to bicycle to our interview, she already has experienced such disability. For several weeks, she had severe peripheral neuropathy, a disorder that to varying degrees affects between one third and one half of persons with HIV disease.[12] She reports:

> It just got harder and harder for me to walk. At one point I was able to crawl on my hands to the bathroom, but I couldn't get from the bathroom floor to the toilet seat. I called all the AIDS organizations—no one could help me. I had a pot and I was able to urinate in the pot. But I just couldn't bring myself to defecate in it. There was someone from the church who came over a couple of times during this time to help me. But I remember one day, because I usually wake up early in the morning, having to defecate, and having to just lay there for hours and crying because I couldn't get to the bathroom.

As their health deteriorates, persons with HIV disease find that they need financial as well as physical assistance from others. Of the thirty-seven people I interviewed, only the three who are professionals and the one who is married to a professional have so far avoided financial ruin.

Even without becoming a burden on others, the drop in their standard of living can seem devastating. Robert, a thirty-eight-year-old former janitor, suggested that we meet at my home rather than his because he was ashamed of the poor quality of his housing. When asked how his financial situation has changed, he replied,

"No Cokes, no tea, no eating out. That sort of thing—doing without. I haven't had any soap in over a year. . . . I've got to save that money for other things, for food especially. . . . I'm not able to shop and buy clothes or anything like that. You feel like you almost are not going to ever be able to build again."

Feelings of shame and low self-esteem increase if individuals must seek government assistance, as most eventually do. David comments that "going into your grocery store, buying food with food stamps, that's embarrassing. It's like you are a degraded part of society now." Moreover, unlike most other developed nations, the United States provides only a minimal standard of living to those on government assistance, forcing many persons with HIV disease to live on incomes below the poverty line. As a result, their standard of living drops precipitously, changing their lifestyles dramatically and further threatening their self-concepts.

Even receiving help from one's family can diminish one's self-esteem. Twenty-two-year-old Jill, for example, now lives with her mother, while her husband, who also has AIDS, lives with his parents. She says:

> I'm having to learn how to accept help. And I've always had a lot of pride. And I've always wanted to work and get it on my own. Now I have to live with my mother, and she has to pay the majority of the bills. And it was very hard to learn how to let her take care [of me], to let her take over. That was really, really hard for me. Or even letting other people help and give without feeling very obligated. You lose a lot of self respect.

Thus, at an age when others are establishing their independence from their families, Jill has had to retreat into dependence and to give up her identity as an independent adult.

The shame persons with HIV disease feel at their dependency and their sense of loss are compounded by the loss of alternative sources of self-esteem and satisfaction. Because of either disability or discrimination, most eventually stop working. Subsequently, they often describe themselves as leading "empty lives" that revolve around the television, their living rooms, and their immediate families. Most importantly, they consider their lives empty because they believe they no longer contribute to society either through their work or in other ways.[13] Clint, for example, had always derived much of his sense of self from his ability and willingness to help his friends and acquaintances. Now he explains through his tears, "I was always one of the people who surrounded myself with people that had problems. And I was always the knight in shining armor. I was always the one saving people . . . and I can't do that anymore."

Taken together, these changes in physical and mental abilities can lead persons with HIV disease to feel that some malevolent, outside force now controls their bodies. David says that having ARC is "like something is alive inside you, and you can't do anything about it. It's like if you were strung out in the desert, and let ants crawl all over you. But it is inside of you." In addition, the nature of this illness can cause individuals to experience at least occasional feelings of dirtiness—of being both contaminated and contaminating. As Brian says, "I have this feeling inside that I'm sort of inferior because I have this dirty nasty disease." Similarly, Carol says, "I'll be laying down in bed or sitting on the couch, and you know you feel the blood circulating. And you think all that blood is so contagious. You know one drop could kill somebody. Which is what it comes down to. I mean they're not going to drop dead immediately but—. And then that makes you feel dirty. It's almost like you can feel it circulating in your veins if you think about it long enough."

These feelings are reinforced daily by the need to adopt anti-contagion measures in such everyday aspects of life as food preparation and house cleaning. Brian describes some of the routine precautions he now takes:

> I don't taste the food that I'm cooking [for the family] and I keep my fingers out of it. If I have some cuts or hangnails or something like that, I don't get in there and mush up meat loaf or whatever. I'll wear gloves. I'm very careful not to cut my finger when I'm slicing tomatoes or something like that. And if I did get blood or something on any food product, I would not allow somebody else to consume it. Of course, I don't cough or sneeze in the kitchen. I wash my hands a lot more than I ever did and I don't pick at my teeth or something like that with my hands. And the bathroom I keep much cleaner than I ever have done. I use Clorox a lot.

Even these precautions seem insufficient to some persons with HIV disease. The general practitioner who diagnosed Susan with AIDS told her that she would die within eighteen months. He instructed her to use only paper plates and paper cups, sterilize all pots and pans, and wash her own clothes with bleach, separately from her family's. Her current doctor has tried to calm her fears that she might infect her family but has been only partially successful. She interrupted our interview at one point to ask why I wasn't scared to be in a room with her, and to ask if I really believed that she could not infect her family. Although she knows that no cases of casual transmission have been documented, she worries that sooner or later it will happen. Consequently, she wonders if her children would be safer if she abandoned them. To calm some of her fears, she now uses a separate set of dishes and washes all dishes and clothes with bleach. These routine actions remind her daily of her illness.

When persons with HIV disease make such changes because of pressure from others rather than by their own choice, the emotional impact can be even greater. Calvin, for example, describing his relationship with a close woman friend, reports that nowadays, "I'm welcome, but there's no physical contact. There's no 'hello,' no greeting, no hug, no anything. The number one rule is I'm not allowed to use her bathroom." When asked how this makes him feel, he replied, "Cheap, degrading, scum, dirty."

Conclusions

All chronic and terminal illnesses threaten the self-concepts of affected individuals.[14] Ill persons frequently experience "failed performances," in which they cannot meet their own expectations regarding who they are and how they should act. They become unable to control their bodies or their minds, care for themselves, present a pleasant physical appearance, or continue their former roles and behaviors. The responses they receive from others following these failed performances and their own reactions to both performance and reaction pressure individuals to replace their former self-concepts with new identities as ill persons who are "set apart" as both different from and inferior to others.[15]

For all these reasons, illness can result in what Charmaz refers to as a "diminished self."[16] As a result, all chronically ill persons must reevaluate their ideas about who they are and develop new ideas to reflect their changed circumstances. As this chapter suggests, however, persons with HIV disease experience especially severe threats to their self-concepts. Persons with diabetes, for example, often view themselves as basically healthy people with sick pancreases. Because HIV disease can affect any bodily organ, however, those who have this illness cannot identify the illness with only one part of their bodies and thus separate the illness from their essential selves. Moreover, because HIV disease impairs mind as well as body, affected individuals cannot cope with their illness as, for example, persons with arthritis do, by stressing that their true selves reside in their intact minds, rather than in their feeble bodies.

To make matters worse, the opportunistic infections that characterize HIV disease can strike at any time. Consequently, individuals have no warning period during which they can bolster their emotional energies to cope with the oncoming onslaught of illness. Moreover, because their level of disabilities can change at any time, persons with HIV disease can never feel that they have achieved equilibrium with their illness and control over their lives.

In addition, because this illness can be transmitted sexually, individuals frequently experience a deep sense of personal pollution and alienation from their sexuality. This is especially problematic for gay and bisexual men, given the preexisting guilt about their sexuality that some feel and the central importance of sexuality in their subcultures.

Persons with HIV disease also find it especially difficult to adjust to their illness because it generally strikes during early adulthood, the age when serious illness is least expected. In contrast, persons who are born ill or become ill as children develop self-concepts early on that incorporate their physical limitations. Those who become ill as older adults are also more prepared because they are at a point in life where they and others expect their abilities to become more limited and their past accomplishments to outshine their future ones. For all these reasons, then, HIV disease can present a devastating blow to the physical, sexual, and intellectual aspects of individuals' self-concepts.

In many ways, living with this illness means coming to terms with loss and, especially, with loss of control. Nevertheless, many persons with HIV disease still manage to feel that they control their lives. Deciding whether to inform health care workers of their diagnosis, for example, can be stressful. Yet the ability to make that decision helps individuals feel that they still have some control over their fates. Similarly, although individuals may have few doctors to choose from, they still will sometimes confront their doctors to demand the kind of care they desire, or, if they have options, seek new doctors who will do so. Most importantly, persons with HIV disease make decisions daily about what they will and will not do to protect their health. These decisions can be diametrically opposed—some, for example, choose to maintain a positive attitude by making plans while others choose to avoid frustration by not doing so. Regardless of what choices individuals make, however, the ability to make choices helps individuals feel in control of their lives and thus helps make life with HIV disease seem worth living.

CHAPTER 6

HIV Disease and Social Relationships

In addition to devastating one's body, HIV disease can also devastate one's social life. As individuals' physical abilities diminish, they can no longer continue their social relationships unaltered. As a result, some relationships end and others become strained. At the same time, the risk of infecting others forces persons with HIV disease to make adjustments in many of their everyday social interactions and can create further emotional distance and stress in relationships. Finally, because HIV disease often reveals or highlights individuals' homosexuality or drug use, and because the illness is itself stigmatized, social relationships may be further strained, as families, friends, lovers, and others reevaluate their moral judgments about ill individuals.

Both their personal experiences and what they learn from the media teach persons with HIV disease that many others condemn them and consider their illness a divine punishment for sin. As a result, they sometimes fear that they will be quarantined or even killed if others learn of their illness. David's worst fears stem from a gruesome story he had heard about the fate of one man who was alleged to have HIV disease:

> I fear that somebody may come in here and beat the shit out of me, or kill me or something like that. . . . It happened in

Florida before I moved from there. A young man was supposedly diagnosed with AIDS and people went in there and ripped his eyes right out of his head. The kid did not have AIDS. He is still in the hospital and doesn't know that he has no eyes in his head. They left him there for dead. They beat him up pretty bad. This was not the first incident, there were four or five of them. . . . There are all kinds of red-necks living across the street, and I'm sure that if they found out a gay person was over here with AIDS, they may decide to get drunk one night and come over and kill the faggot.

Similarly, whenever police helicopters fly overhead during the night, Susan has nightmares that they are coming to get her. Such fears of social reactions are so strong that Brent says he would rather die than be cured and have to live the rest of his life with the stigma of having once had HIV disease. These feelings lead individuals to describe themselves as the modern world's equivalent of lepers.

Family Relationships

Following diagnosis with a serious illness or other similar trauma, most persons will turn to their families for support. For persons with HIV disease, however, this coping strategy is fraught with dangers. Knowing that so many Americans fear or despise those who have this illness, many worry how their families will react to news of their diagnosis. This is particularly true if their diagnosis will expose or emphasize their gayness or drug use. Dick, for example, is a twenty-seven-year-old computer operator with ARC, whose parents live in a small midwestern town. He believes he has a good relationship with them, but has never told them that he is gay. When asked how he thinks they will react to news of his diagnosis, he says, "You just can't predict. They might find it so disgusting that you'll basically lose them. They'll be gone. Or they'll go through the adjustment period and not mind. You really don't know."

Other persons with HIV disease assume, based on statements their relatives have made previously, that their response will be unsympathetic. Tom, for example, considers his father "very homophobic" and his mother "very religious," and so was afraid how they might respond to news of his diagnosis. When he started experiencing serious health problems, however, he decided that he needed to tell them. He changed his mind when, as he describes, "I think of it almost as an anticipation of the news that they kind of went into some rather insensitive things about Rock Hudson and about how [it is] the 'just desserts' for the homosexual community that AIDS has come up and so on." Tom has decided not to tell his family of his illness unless it becomes unavoidable. Dick, meanwhile, like several others whose families live out of state, has decided to wait until he can tell them in person.

Others do not tell their families because they cannot deal with their own feelings of shame. Calvin's sense of shame had led him to sever all contact with his ex-wife (whom he still loved) and his young children when he started having gay relationships years ago. Despite the knowledge that he is dying, he has decided to continue this silence. As he explains, "I haven't seen my kids for almost twelve years and when AIDS came down, I didn't know how to handle it. How do you tell your kids two thousand miles away that you're not only homosexual, but you're dying from a killer disease, the 'gay plague' as I call it? How do you do that? How do you explain a lifetime in a thirty-minute telephone conversation? So I chose not to."

Although hiding their illness protects individuals from rejection, it creates other problems. Those who do not tell their relatives deprive themselves of emotional or practical support that they might otherwise receive from their families. In addition, relationships necessarily become strained when persons with HIV disease cannot discuss some of the most important issues in their lives. For these reasons, most eventually tell their families of their diagnoses.

The experiences of persons with HIV disease who reveal their illness suggests that fears of rejection are warranted. This is especially true for those who are gay. Almost every gay man I interviewed who has told his family reports that at least one family member has ended contact with him, and a few report that all relatives have done so. This rejection largely occurs because diagnosis with HIV disease reinforces families' preexisting repugnance at homosexuality. Families that always had questioned the morality of homosexuality may interpret an individual's illness as divine punishment and proof that they should never have tolerated such behavior. For example, before he became ill, Jeremy's fundamentalist Christian family did not know he was gay. By forcing him to reveal his sexual orientation, HIV disease has, in Jeremy's words, "put a wedge" between him and his family. So long as he continues his "sinful" lifestyle, his family feels that they should not help him with his health and financial problems. He still speaks with his parents, but has stopped talking to his sister because he cannot abide her constant admonitions to "repent" and to "confess sin."

Because HIV disease makes individuals' homosexuality more concrete to their families, even those whose families previously seemed to accept their lifestyles may experience rejection once the diagnoses become known. Just as pregnancy forces parents to recognize that their daughter is not just living with a man but having sex with him, diagnosis with HIV disease can force families to recognize that their son or brother is not simply gay in some abstract way, but actually has sex with other men. As a result, families that, despite their moral qualms, once had tolerated their son's or brother's homosexuality may no longer do so. For example, before he was diagnosed, Hugh would routinely bring his lover home with him. His mother had always acted courteously toward his lover and seemed at least to tolerate his homosexuality. When he informed her of his diagnosis, however, she told him, "I think your lifestyle is vulgar. I have never understood it. I've never accepted it. . . . Your lifestyle repulses me." She subsequently refused to let him in her house or even to help him obtain medical insurance.

Families may also reject persons with HIV disease because they fear that they, too, will be stigmatized should the diagnosis become known. Calvin has been abandoned by every member of his large and formerly close-knit family, all of whom knew of and apparently accepted his homosexuality in the past:

> This is back in a farming town in Indiana. It's like they would die, I mean literally die, if I went to that town and walked down that street and neighbors saw me. Even though the neighbors didn't know that I had AIDS, they would think that the neighbors could tell from the way I walked. They're scared and they've become very selfish of their own feelings and hurts because they have to live in that community. In a few months I'll be dead, but they have to live there the rest of their lives and they're not about to be disgraced.

Compared to the gay men I interviewed, the women have experienced few such difficulties. The main difference is that their families' reactions to HIV disease are not as confounded by repugnance at stigmatized behavior. Seven of the fourteen women had been infected through heterosexual intercourse or blood transfusions. Although the remaining seven had been infected through drug use, only two, Carol and Jeanne, were still using drugs at the time of diagnosis. The rest were "reformed" addicts who now profess their belief in the virtues of a drug-free life. None of the women's families of origin rejected them or considered HIV disease a just punishment, although Carrie has not told her fundamentalist Christian family of her diagnosis because she assumes they will consider her illness a deserved punishment for nonmarital sex. In addition, although neither Carol's nor Susan's families consider HIV disease a just punishment for their drug use, their in-laws do.

Even when families do not overtly reject their ill relatives, however, their behavior can still create a sense of stigma. This can happen when families either hide the illnesses altogether or tell others that their son, daughter, brother, or sister has some other, less stigmatized, illness. In some cases, parents or siblings additionally ordered the people I interviewed not to tell other relatives of their illness. This imposed secrecy places heavy burdens on those who subsequently must "live a lie." It also forces them to recognize how deeply their families either fear the stigma of HIV disease or resent or are embarrassed by their gayness or drug use.

Families can further reinforce a sense of stigma by adopting extreme and medically unwarranted anticontagion measures. Walter's relatives, for example, bring their own sheets whenever they visit. Other families refuse to allow persons with HIV disease to touch any food, share their bathrooms, or come closer than an arm's length away. Jack, for example, is a twenty-nine-year-old salesperson whose Mormon family believes HIV disease is a just punishment for his former gay activities. Initially, his family "wouldn't come in the room unless they had gloves and a mask and they wouldn't touch me. . . . [And] for a time I couldn't go over to somebody's house for dinner. And they still use paper plates [when I eat there]." Even those persons with HIV disease who believe such precautions are necessary miss their lost physical warmth and intimacy and feel stigmatized, isolated, and contaminated. Such behavior, however, may be becoming less common as the general public become more educated about HIV disease. Unlike the men and women interviewed in 1986 and 1987, all the women interviewed in 1989 reported that, once the initial shock was over and their families received some basic biological information about HIV disease, no family member rejected them out of fear of infection.

Relationships also suffer when families either deny their relatives' illness or constantly focus on it. Sharon is a thirty-five-year old laboratory technician with ARC whose mother does both:

> My mother has not accepted the fact that I am infected. She's had a very difficult time dealing with it. We can't even talk about it. She's, "Oh, you'll be here at Christmas." And I may not be here, you know, because I could get sick. . . . As long as I'm doing well then everything is okay. But if I'm not feeling well, she doesn't want to discuss it.

And:

> She just tries to smother me. Like every time, like if I have a headache or if I'm not feeling well and don't want to go out. "You're not sick are you?" She just constantly reminds me that I'm infected.

Both behaviors are difficult for persons with HIV disease and both can create additional emotional stress for individuals and strain in their relationships with others.

Yet despite all these potential sources of stress, HIV disease can also heal, rather than create, family divisions. Dennis, for example, at fifty-seven, is the oldest person I interviewed. He has never gotten along with his father, whom he considered a cold and selfish man. Since becoming ill, however, they have gotten considerably closer. As he describes, "There's the verbal 'I love you.' There's the letters. One of the nicest things that's ever happened to me . . . is my father sent me a personal card. In the inside he wrote 'God bless you. I love you son.' . . . It meant the world to me." Sarah, a thirty-year-old bookkeeper who contracted AIDS following a relationship with a man who had hemophilia, has had a similar experience. In the past, she had only known that her parents loved her because they bought her things. She says, "I was getting materialistic things and that wasn't what I wanted. What I wanted was to be held and for them to tell me they loved me and do things with me and stuff like that. . . . From the time I've been diagnosed, my mom has been either holding my hand or hugging me or letting me know that she loves me. The same way with my father. It's really changed them." Others report that their families now telephone, visit, or write much more often than before.

Diagnosis can also bring families together by ending previous sources of conflict. Either to preserve their own health, to protect others from infection, or because they lose interest in sex once diagnosed with a deadly, sexually transmitted disease, gay men who have HIV disease may cease all sexual activities. Similar motives may prompt those who became infected through drug use to abstain from drugs. In addition, concern about their health can motivate individuals to stop smoking tobacco and drinking alcohol. As a result, families that previously had disapproved of their relatives' lifestyles may stop considering their relatives either sinful or emotionally sick, even if these individuals continue to consider themselves gay or to desire drugs. Consequently, some persons with HIV disease achieve a new acceptance from relatives who attach less stigma to their illness than to homosexuality or drug use.

HIV disease can also unify families as they struggle to confront a hostile world. This is most obvious in Jill's case. Jill's husband, brother-in-law, and nephew all are hemophiliacs and all have HIV disease, as did another nephew who recently died. To cope with the physical and social consequences of HIV disease, the family has become tighter-knit than before. Everyone in the family has had to learn about the disease and become accustomed to dealing with people who are infected. As a result, although HIV disease is a tragedy and a source of stigma from the outside world, it has strengthened rather than weakened relationships within the family.

Lovers and Spouses

Having HIV disease also significantly alters relationships with lovers and spouses. At the time of diagnosis, seven of the twenty-three men and eleven of the fourteen women were married or in ongoing relationships with lovers. Because these lovers and spouses all had helped in the decision to seek medical help, the individuals I interviewed could not hide news of their diagnosis from them, as some had from their families. Consequently, all eighteen immediately told their husbands or lovers of their diagnosis.

In response to this news, five of the eighteen (two men and three women) were abandoned by their partners. For example, Marshall's lover left him soon after his diagnosis. He reports, "The guy that I was seeing at that time, he didn't want to deal with it anymore. It was to the point he called me up one time and he said, 'I've been seeing somebody for three weeks now'—which [meant] he was seeing him while he and I were seeing still seeing each other. And he made the comment, he goes, 'And he's healthy.' " In addition to the five whose partners left, one individual left her partner. Once Sharon learned that her husband had known he was infected with HIV but had continued to have unprotected sex with her without even telling her that he and therefore she was at risk, she ordered him to leave and never return.

The remaining twelve lovers and husbands did not abandon their partners. Four were infected with HIV and one, who did not know his HIV status, assumed he was infected. As a result, these individuals had no reason to fear initial infection (although some did fear reinfection) and less reason to fear stigma. They thus had less reason than others to end these relationships. Another six who were not infected and one who had no idea whether or not he was infected also chose to stay with their partners.

As is the case with family relationships, some relationships with lovers or spouses improve as a result of diagnosis with HIV disease. When one or both partners is infected, both may recognize how much the other means to them and how much it would hurt to lose the other. For example, before he learned he had HIV disease, Jeremy had resisted making any commitment to his lover, wanting to wait until they had known each other for at least a year before moving in together or in any other way signifying that this might be a special relationship. After his diagnosis, he realized that he wanted to share his life with this man. Now, according to Jeremy, "The time we spend together is a lot more meaningful. And it's not always trying to pack a lot into it. It's more quality time now. We care more. The care that we take in cooking our meals for each other. There's a lot more put into it. There's a lot more love there than there was." They have since decided to have their relationship blessed in their church, as a substitute for the marriage that they cannot obtain under the law. Similarly, Carrie says, "My boyfriend's and my relationship is twice as good as it was before.

He was totally noncommittal. Wishy-washy. A pain in the butt. And the other night, he said, . . . 'They could take my car. And they could take my house.' And he said, 'You know, they can take all that . . ., but they can't take us. They can't take the love that we have.' So things are better for me than they were before."

The mere survival of a relationship is not necessarily a good thing, however. Keith, for example, is a thirty-five-year old mechanic who has ARC. He began his current relationship shortly after his lover of eighteen years died in a car accident. His current lover is fifteen years his junior, and shares few of his values or interests. Nevertheless, Keith and Andy stay together. As Keith explains, "I think it [ARC] has probably brought me to a realization that, I hate to sound crass, but, hey, you better settle for what you've got, because now this is all you're gonna get. I mean, what am I going to do now? If I choose to leave Andy, what am I going to do now? Am I going to take an ad out in a gay paper somewhere saying, 'Person with AIDS seeking someone else with AIDS?' I couldn't do that." Thus, although Keith feels "trapped" in this relationship, he has not left it. Conversely, other individuals wonder whether their partners stay with them simply out of loyalty or pity rather than love. The resulting doubts and constant need for reassurance can place great strain on relationships.

HIV disease can damage relationships in other ways as well. Although neither Mary's husband nor Susan's has threatened to leave, both sometimes seethe with anger and doubts about how their wives became infected. Because Mary's husband had not known that she had used drugs prior to the marriage, he sometimes finds her drug use difficult to believe, and wonders if she didn't really become infected through an affair. Similarly, Susan's husband had used drugs with her but is not himself infected. As a result, he wonders if she betrayed him sexually, and is almost equally angry at the thought that she shared needles with someone else (an activity that has quasi-sexual meaning among drug users).

Relationships also suffer because of the financial strain the illness causes. Both persons with HIV disease and their partners may resent the former's increasing financial dependence and deplore the inequality that dependence creates in their relationships. At the same time, persons with HIV disease may feel guilty about impoverishing their spouses or tying them to disliked jobs for the income or medical insurance. As Mary says, "I'm seeing him not being able to go on, and I feel I'm holding him back [in terms of] his job, his life, everything. He can't do anything. He can't plan anything. It's not fair. And he says it doesn't bother him, but I know it does."

Other problems develop when partners, like parents, either become overprotective or deny the seriousness of the illness. Susan's husband, for example, angrily refuses to discuss anything having to do with death, dying, or sickness. Jeremy's lover gets upset whenever Jeremy does not do his share of the housework, forgetting or denying that Jeremy might have been too sick to do so. Similarly, Calvin says:

> It has created a block, a stake that's been driven through the friendship and relationship that I have with my roommate who was my lover for ten years. . . . He cares so much about me that the thought of losing me is more than he can handle. So he cannot deal with my AIDS. He will not accept my AIDS. To him there's been a mistake. The tests need to be run over. I'm fine. If I get up and walk from my chair to the kitchen and get a glass of pop, in his mind I'm cured, I'm well. So it's very hard to live under those circumstances, because, like I said earlier, I'm sick, I'm very sick. But when he's around I have to pretend that I'm okay and play a game and be an actor simply because he hurts worse for me than I hurt for myself. We're that close and he can't deal with it. I'm not allowed to talk about it. I'm not allowed to grunt, be in pain, change my life. My life has to be exactly the way it was before I was diagnosed because that's where his head is at. If I slip and get angry and make a statement about, "Oh, fuck it! I'm going to be dead in a few months from AIDS anyhow," if he is sit-

ting in the kitchen, he's gone. I see nothing but his dust to his bedroom with the door closed because he won't deal with this. He won't face this. So AIDS has changed my life in that respect, because I can't be what I want to be and that's just sick. I have to continually perform. And I get tired, but I can't let my guard down, for his sake. So it has changed our relationship. We don't talk anymore. He won't talk to me for fear I'm going to say something about AIDS. He comes home after I'm in bed and leaves before I get up because he doesn't want to face me for fear I'm going to say something about AIDS. He's that frightened . . . for me. I've lost a friend.

Another arena for conflict between persons with HIV disease and their partners is sex. Some who have this illness still desire sexual contact but find that their partners do not, either because the partners fear infection with HIV, or, if already infected, fear that they could become more ill if they are reinfected. In other cases, the healthy partners desire sexual activity but the ill partners do not. In these circumstances, the ill partners may feel obliged to simulate interest to please their lovers or husbands. Debbie says:

There are times when he comes up and he's making eyes and I just want to tell him, "Leave me alone, I feel like crap." But I don't dare ever say that, because I'm afraid if I say no, well, he's just going to leave. So I deal with that. And we've talked about it, and I know he doesn't feel like that. But I can't make that fear go away, and I can't rationalize it away. So I say yes. And so then he's like, "Well, that was like being with a beached whale." You know, I don't feel like two cents.

Susan's situation is even worse, for her husband has said he will leave her if she denies him sexual access and will sue her for child custody if she ever leaves him. Her descriptions of their sexual interactions sound little short of rape, especially given her 80-pound frame and his 220 pounds. Such situations force individuals to question their former ideas about themselves, their partners, and the nature of their relationships.

Those whose partners are themselves ill face a different set of problems. Karen is a twenty-seven-year-old waitress who is infected with HIV. She has had few health problems so far, but her husband has AIDS. Neither of them has any relatives in the state, so she bears sole responsibility for caring for her husband and their uninfected toddler:

> It's physically demanding. . . . I'm worried, scared. It's been very difficult, because usually I work a 4:00 to 10:00 P.M. Sometimes I work a 5:30 P.M. to 12:00 or 1:00 shift. I get home, and he's usually still awake, and at that time of the night he's usually in his worst pain or having fever. . . . He's afraid to sleep a lot of nights because he's afraid he's just not going to wake up because of pneumocystis. And he does have bronchial asthma. . . . And I've tried to stay up with him because he's afraid. You know, I want to be there for support. And when nine, ten o'clock rolls around, the baby wakes up and I might get three or four hours of sleep, if I'm lucky. Sometimes I go for months solid like that. And after a while up at work I'm just like, "Slap me so I can even function."

Walter, a thirty-seven-year-old clerical worker, never got the chance to take care of the man he loved. Shortly before the first interview, Walter had fallen in love with another man who had the same illness. To protect themselves emotionally should one of them become sicker, they had decided to live together but not to become lovers. At the follow-up interview, Walter describes what happened:

> We had got a brand-new apartment and everything, and I didn't even fix that up because I was waiting for Phil to come

home. He only got to stay one night there; he went to his
folks and his mom. That was rough on me because there was
nothing I could do for him. Every day was bad for him. His
mother wanted to do it all, and I really couldn't do it either
because I would have gotten too involved and sick.

Nevertheless, he soon found himself in the hospital, along with
Phil, who was seriously ill and in constant pain:

> Everything was happening too fast. And I was worried about
> Phil, Phil was worried about me. He came and saw me twice
> in the hospital, and he was in his wheelchair. I cried when he
> left both times, and it's like he gave me this little wave. We
> couldn't talk, even when he was sick. We couldn't talk [be-
> cause] someone was always around. . . . The only time we
> really got to talk was when he spent the night, the one
> night. . . . That night, I says, "Phil, I want you to either get
> better or die. I don't want you to keep going through this."

When Phil went into the hospital for the last time:

> Phil didn't want anybody to be upset over him being sick, so
> everybody was trying to be strong. Soon as he got to the room,
> I ran to the bathroom and went to a men's stall and just broke
> down. I think that was almost my goodbye to him.

For Walter, love seems to have brought pain outweighing its joys.
    A main issue for those who either are not in relationships at
the time of diagnosis or are subsequently abandoned by their partners is whether to seek new relationships. Because of the potential
for transmitting HIV to another during sexual activity, and because
of the potential for rejection if one suggests entering a sexual relationship, fourteen men and three women have sworn off sexual relationships altogether, despite the sense of loss this has created for

them. A few of these men, however, have had sex with anonymous partners on rare occasions when their fears and guilt had led them to drink until too drunk to make any conscious decisions.

For those who choose to enter new relationships, deciding whether to inform their lovers that they are infected presents a major ethical dilemma. The issues are complex, for they must decide both how to protect themselves from stigma and how to protect others from infection.

Of the remaining eight, six always tell their lovers that they are infected and two do not. The six who tell believe it is unfair to risk exposing someone to infection without their knowledge. In addition, one of these six, Sally, will only have sex with men who are also infected with HIV. (However, she had shared a needle on one recent occasion with an unsuspecting partner because she had wanted the drug too much to care if she infected him.) In contrast, Dick and Marshall believe that they need not disclose their diagnoses as long as they restrict themselves to activities unlikely to transmit the virus. Besides, they argue, disclosure is unnecessary because most gay or bisexual men already have been exposed to the virus. As Dick says, "The level of infection in that group is so high that if, in fact, *you* are careful not to exchange body fluids to *them,* then their level of risk out of this encounter is much lower than what they probably did the week before. And they found *that* acceptable."

Relationships with Friends

Similar issues surface in talking to persons with HIV disease about their relationships with their friends. Again, individuals must decide whether to disclose news of their diagnosis to friends, some of whom do not know that they are gay or use drugs. And again, just as when individuals do not tell their families, those who do not tell their friends both forfeit any emotional support they might otherwise have received and place strains on their relationships. Moreover, although the families of persons with HIV disease often live at some geographic distance from them, friends typically live considerably closer. As a result, individuals more often must lie or obfuscate when talking to friends than when talking to relatives.

Having to field questions and remarks from friends who have a mistaken notion about what is happening in their lives can create considerable strain. Debbie, for example, has told most of her friends that she has cancer. As a result, she often has to listen and respond to remarks from friends who mean to reassure her about how cancer can be cured. As she explains, "I have people calling me all the time and telling me up-to-the-minute reports on cancer research because that's what they think I have. And it's just like, oh, I'm so sick of this! I just want to take out a front-page ad and tell everybody I have AIDS so please leave me alone!" Thus, secretiveness itself can create emotional stress for persons with HIV disease. As Morgan, a thirty-eight-year-old nurse, says, "I want to tell. I'm not used to hiding everything from everybody. . . . . I'm a basically honest person, and I don't like to lie."

These stresses pressure individuals to tell their friends of their diagnosis. Recognizing the dangers, though, they devise strategies for deciding both whom to tell and when to tell of their illnesses. For example, Marshall, who has been abandoned by several close friends, says, "I used to tell people up front about my diagnosis, but I don't any more. I let them get to know me, because I really want them to get to know me before they pass judgment on me." Others talk to friends about the epidemic of HIV disease, make up stories about friends who are infected, or discuss their work for community organizations that deal with HIV disease to gauge their friends' reactions. They then decide if it is safe to disclose their diagnosis.

Following disclosure, some friendships end immediately. Typically, persons with HIV disease report that some friends "are very supportive, come around, enjoy coming over here, whatever. But most of them have backed off." For example, Marshall says that when his best friend learned of his diagnosis, "He couldn't get me out of his apartment fast enough." Other friendships also suffered: "It was to the point [my friends] didn't even want to be in the same room with me. . . . It was just like 'don't call us, we'll call you. . . .' They stopped returning calls. When I would see them out [at bars], they would see me coming, and they would head out in the other direction."

As is the case with families, however, disclosure sometimes strengthens relationships. Sharon believes her relationships with the four friends she has told have become better. She says:

> I think we finally realized that we are very good friends. We just took it for granted that, yeah, we're friends, and we go out and have dinner together. Now it's like every day I talk to those four people, because they're all at work. Even if just to say, "Hi, how're you doing?" Every day we go out of our way to talk to each other, you know, because they want to keep tabs on me. It's like my little secret force I have at work. And if I don't see them then they want to know why. "Why didn't you come down and see me?" They get very angry if I don't see them every day. And that makes me feel really good.

Similar experiences led Tom, whose family has told him that HIV disease is "just desserts" for homosexuals, to conclude "that family are those people . . . you can really love and trust and care for" and not necessarily one's blood relations.

Even when relationships survive news of their diagnosis, however, the dynamics of those relationships can change for the worse. Because they worry about the health of the person who is ill, friends will often change their behavior in a variety of ways that they believe are in the individuals' best interests—asking persons with HIV disease about their dietary restrictions before inviting them for dinner, or trying not to tire them out by keeping them up too late. As Marshall describes:

> Some people try to bend over backward to do things for you. They almost consider it like you're a cripple or something like

that. You know, "Well, let me help you with that. Are you sure you can lift this?" And they're just like so overconsiderate.

Similarly, friends can try to protect persons with HIV disease from emotional stress. Jill says:

> The thing that kind of makes me angry with my friends is they don't want to call and tell me their problems anymore. They don't want to talk about it. They don't want to dump on me, you know. And I keep telling them, "Hey, misery loves company," so they'll call me up. Sometimes they walk on eggshells around me. But I'm very honest and open about it and say, "Will you just knock it off?" You know? "Call me if you need to talk to me because I don't want to be treated any different or any special."

Such behavior rankles because it makes individuals feel that they are no longer equal partners in these friendships. Instead, they feel "pointed out and set apart."

Despite their annoyance at being treated differently, however, persons with HIV disease themselves must make many changes in their lifestyles to protect their health. Sharon, for example, describes her life as "very tunnelled." She says:

> There are certain things that have made my life very, very hard to live in. I mean, because I don't go out to the bars, or go out with my friends when they say, "Let's go out and have a drink." I don't go because the chances of me wanting a drink, and the effects it will have on me, I just don't go.

As their illness progresses, individuals become physically unable to participate in social activities such as sports, drinking, and dancing. Brent, who has AIDS, says:

> I can't get out and do things. I can't work and meet people, so there's a great sense of loneliness in it. The times when I'm

feeling my best is during the daytime when most people are at their work, school, whatever. Of course at nighttime when they're all free to go out and party and whatnot, I'm beginning to wind down. There are fewer and fewer times when I can make it out with them. There's a real sense of loneliness. The TV and my parents are my best friends these days.

As they withdraw from the social activities that had nourished their friendships, persons with HIV disease and their friends find they have less and less in common. Although some friendships can survive these changes, others cannot. Thus, whether because of stigma or ill health, the social circles of persons with HIV disease narrow significantly.

Relationships with Children

Both having and not having children can create problems for persons with HIV disease. A man who is infected with HIV cannot biologically father children without risking infecting the mother. A woman who is infected has between a 20 and a 50 percent chance of infecting any babies she bears, through a mechanism that remains unclear. As a result, both men and women often decide that they should not have children. Jill, for example, had accidentally become pregnant after learning that she was infected with HIV. She had seen her young nephew sicken and die of AIDS and knew that any child of hers might meet the same fate. In addition, she assumed both that her own health would suffer if she became pregnant and that she and her husband would both die soon and leave any child of theirs an orphan. As a result, she decided to have an abortion. She carried through on this decision, even though she had to brave antiabortion demonstrators at the clinic.

Even when deciding not to have children seems the only logical choice, it still can carry a heavy emotional cost. This seems especially true for women. None of the men mentioned their childlessness as an issue, but half the childless women regarded this as a major source of grief in their life. Jill, for example, still believes that she made the right decision, but nevertheless expresses great sorrow over the need to make that choice. Similarly, for months after she learned she was infected, Sarah cried every time she saw a baby food commercial on television.

Persons with HIV disease who already have children describe a different set of problems. On the one hand, individuals may benefit from a new closeness with their children, as they discover how much they mean to each other and consciously choose to spend time together. On the other hand, they may worry that those relationships are becoming too close, as they find it increasingly difficult to let their children have their own lives away from the household. In addition, relationships with children can become strained if they, like parents or spouses, deny the reality of their parents' illness—refusing, for example, to take over some of their parents' chores because their parents "aren't really that sick." As the illness progresses, relationships with children can suffer further, as parents become unable to play with their children or interact in ways the children find satisfying or meaningful. This is especially true if they are too young to understand why their parents have withdrawn.

Having children can also increase stress for persons with HIV disease by forcing them to confront their own mortality in ways that others who have this illness can avoid. Many persons with HIV disease defer making a will because they do not want to acknowledge the likelihood of their own deaths. Those who have children, however, do not have that luxury, for they must make guardianship and financial arrangements for them. In addition, although all persons with HIV disease grieve over the loss of their own future, that loss seems more concrete for those who have children. Having children gives individuals a very specific sense of what they will be missing—seeing their children grow up, graduate, marry, or the like. Sharon says:

> It makes me crazy some days to know that I may not be able to see [my daughter] graduate from high school, and go to college, and get married and give me grandkids. But that's

just something I really don't think about because there's nothing I can do about it. I live day by day. I can't think about the future, because it just makes me very depressed, and I don't allow myself to get depressed.

Similarly, regrets over their own death are amplified by feelings of guilt about leaving their children behind. As Karen says:

If I wouldn't have had a child, I don't think it would have affected me as much. I think I would have been able to accept it a little bit better. But having a child, it's like, you know, you want to be there for them. You don't want to leave them an orphan or whatever. That was the toughest thing.

Perhaps the only burden that persons with HIV disease can endure that is worse than knowing that they will leave their children orphans is knowing that they have contributed to their children's deaths. Of those I interviewed, only Carol was in this position, having infected her baby before birth. Carol seems overwhelmed by her sense of guilt, grief, and shame. To cope with these feelings, she has distanced herself emotionally from her baby, although not from her older, uninfected, child. She says, "There really isn't even that bond like there is with my two-year-old. It's almost like he isn't mine." She feels that she has "purposely" distanced herself because of her sense of guilt and inadequacy as a mother for doing this to her baby. As she explains, "Because there's no way around it. I did it. I can't pass the buck to anybody else. There's no other excuse. I did it. And I don't know, there's just no bond. I'm not even sure if I love him. I would kill for him, don't get me wrong. He's my child. There isn't anything I wouldn't do for him. But there's just not that feeling. When I hold him, he's like somebody else's child."

Work Relationships

By the time individuals receive diagnoses of HIV disease, many are physically incapable of working. Others, faced with catastrophic medical bills, must quit their jobs to qualify for state-financed medical assistance.

Those who continue working risk stigma and discrimination if others learn of their illness. Although most courts have ruled that persons with HIV disease are disabled and thus qualify for protection under antidiscrimination laws,[1] in practice, employers can fire persons with HIV disease with impunity because few have the time, money, or stamina to sue successfully. As a result, individuals may decide not to tell their employers and co-workers of their illness.

Although hiding one's illness can help protect individuals from discrimination and rejection, it carries a high price. Those who hide their illnesses from their employers may lose their jobs when they cannot explain their increased absences and decreased productivity. In addition, they occasionally must endure uncensored remarks from others about how HIV disease "serves those queers right" or is a just punishment for "sluts" and addicts. Moreover, they may feel that they cannot respond without risking exposure. For example, after one of Debbie's co-workers died of AIDS, she decided always to eat lunch alone to avoid hearing the "crap" her other co-workers were saying about him and so she would not "give herself away" by her reactions. Debbie subsequently quit her job because of declining health and because she could not tolerate the way the one friend and co-worker she had told rejected her. Similarly, Mitch, a thirty-three-year-old salesperson, describes his problems at his former place of employment. He says, "I was at my desk and three secretaries telling AIDS jokes were standing right behind me. It cut and it hurt. I grit my teeth and said nothing. . . . [Occasionally] I try and slide in a little bit of education . . . but I don't push it to the point where they go, 'How come he knows so much?' "

To avoid questions about why they don't find AIDS jokes humorous, some persons with HIV disease feel obliged to join in the laughter. Karen still works as a waitress, but has not told anyone at work of her diagnosis. A few months ago, her boss fired a gay co-worker on the grounds that fear of HIV disease would keep customers away from any establishment with gay waiters, healthy or not. As a result, Karen is careful to censor her responses whenever co-workers joke about HIV disease. As she explains, "I get very angry [but] I don't say anything. I try to just control it because I know I have a very expressive face. My emotions show. So what I try to do is just like, 'Ha, ha, that's funny, you know.' And I turn around and go, 'Grrrr!' And I just walk out of there as fast as I can."

Only Keith, Sharon, and Jill, all of whom work for major corporations, have both told their employers of their diagnosis and kept their jobs. None of these three, however, has told his or her current supervisors; Sharon did tell a former supervisor and was forced to change to a different unit because of discrimination. Moreover, only Sharon has told any co-workers. Nevertheless, Jill still experiences hostility and stigma from co-workers who know that her husband has hemophilia and suspect that he is infected with HIV.

With the exception of these three, all the others who disclosed their illness were either fired immediately, demoted, or forced to quit by co-workers or employers who made their situations intolerable. Jeremy, for example, used to work as a tailor. Initially, his co-workers responded well, taking only reasonable precautions such as not sharing drinking glasses. As time passed, however, their responses grew less rational. As he describes: "Then little things happened. . . . If a pin came from [my department] they would immediately throw it away because [they thought] if they poked themselves, they could get AIDS. . . . [Then they developed] a list of things for me to do at the end of the day like wipe down the scissors and the table and everything that I touched with a weak solution of ten-to-one [bleach]. . . . With all that happening, I kind of lost the desire to work." Shortly thereafter, he quit his job. Although he appeared to have a strong legal case, he decided he did not have the energy, funds, or time to sue.

The only person who has decided to sue is Carrie. A career military officer, Carrie learned that she was infected with HIV as a result of the military's routine screening. She immediately was de-

moted from a job she loved to a job located forty-five minutes farther away that paid $375 less per month. Moreover, she was
informed that as soon as she develops any opportunistic infections,
or her T-cell counts (a sign of immune system functioning) drop
below a certain point, she will be dismissed from the service. Once
dismissed, she will receive considerably lower disability benefits
than had she contracted some other illness. Because Carrie has not
yet experienced any health problems due to HIV, she still has the
physical strength to pursue a court case. In addition, because she
was infected through heterosexual intercourse with a lover, rather
than through some more socially unacceptable activity, she has a
strong sense of righteousness and is indignant at the treatment she
has received. As a result, she also has the emotional strength needed
to pursue a case. Carrie has met with representatives from various
civil rights organizations and plans to file suit soon.

The stigma against persons with HIV disease in the workplace is so strong that it can even affect individuals who are only
suspected of being infected. Recall that Grace is still unsure
whether she is infected with HIV (see Chapter 4). At our second
meeting, by which time she had received two negative ELISA tests
and two indeterminate Western Blot tests, Grace said,

> Although the longer this goes on, the better the odds that I
> am negative, the longer it goes on and I continue to talk out
> about my status, the more I am treated as if I am positive. It's
> really ironic. . . . I am actively job hunting now. I am not
> totally comfortable with putting down on my résumé [the
> community organization that deals with HIV disease where
> she had been working part-time]. But otherwise, how do I
> explain what I have been doing for the last year? I hadn't
> thought about it before, but someone had mentioned it to me.
> And I have been so public about my status, doing interviews
> and speaking on panels. I am not applying for anything work-
> ing with kids, even though I'd like to, because I don't want
> to have to deal with the possibility of discrimination.

These fears seem justified, given the reactions she has experienced so far: Grace has been threatened with legal suit by a former lover, who fears that he will become stigmatized if she continues to speak out, and by the day care center where she used to work, which fears that parents will withdraw their children if they learn that a former worker may be infected with HIV.

Conclusions

In many ways, the changes in social relationships experienced by persons with HIV disease parallel those experienced by others who have chronic or terminal illnesses. All illnesses can result in strained relationships because of their associated physical, sexual, financial, and emotional consequences. And all have the potential for strengthening relationships as individuals realize how much they mean to each other.

Nevertheless, the impact of HIV disease on social relationships differs from the impact of other illnesses in two major ways. First, many persons with HIV disease must cope with not only their illness but that of their spouses, lovers, or children. The resulting guilt, depression, sense of loss, and physical stress are thus considerably greater than they otherwise would be. Second, because HIV disease is contagious, deforming, fatal, imperfectly understood, and associated with groups that already experience stigma, no other contemporary physical illness carries such severe stigma.

Stigma seems least problematic for those whom most Americans consider to be "innocent" victims of HIV disease—children infected by their mothers, wives infected by their husbands, and men and women infected by blood transfusions. Even these individuals can experience considerable stigma, however. Within intimate relationships, stigma seems to be greatest when illness is connected to homosexuality. The stigma experienced by the women who had used drugs (including those who were still using at the time of diagnosis) was on average far milder. In addition, in describing the reactions of others to their diagnosis, the three gay men who had used intravenous drugs consistently referred to the impact that their homosexuality had on their relationships but did not mention any impact of their drug use. Disclosure of homosexuality seems to result in a release of deep-seated repugnance, fear, and anger that, even in this age of "zero tolerance," disclosure of drug use does not.

CHAPTER 7

Making a Life with HIV Disease

To individuals who first learn that they have HIV disease, the problems this will bring can seem overwhelming. For some men and women, these problems remain overwhelming until death overtakes them. Others, however, over time, develop strategies to make living with HIV disease more manageable despite the physical, social, and emotional problems it causes. These strategies help individuals cope with the fear and the reality of social stigma, the changes in their social relationships, the impact of illness on their bodies, and their impending deaths.

Avoiding Stigma

A central part of having HIV disease is the experience of stigma. Stigma is a concern during all phases of the illness, from before diagnosis, when individuals must evaluate the risk of discrimination if they get tested for HIV, to the time when death seems inevitable and they must cope with the possibility of discrimination by funeral directors. As a result, one of the basic tasks persons with HIV disease confront is learning to avoid or reduce stigma.

A basic stratagem used by persons with HIV disease, as by those who have other stigmatized illnesses, is to hide the nature of

128

their illness.[1] Hiding can begin at the time of diagnosis, if individuals and their doctors decide to provide false or misleading information to government disease registries or health insurance companies, and can occur in all social relationships.

Persons with HIV disease use a variety of methods to hide their illnesses. Jeremy routinely transfers his zidovudine pills to an unmarked bottle because he fears that others might recognize the drug as one used to treat HIV disease. Those whose tongues show the telltale whitish spots of candidiasis (an infection that frequently accompanies this illness) close their mouths partially while smiling or talking. Others select clothing or use makeup to hide their emaciation or skin problems.

Most importantly, individuals learn to gauge how sick they look on any given day. Whenever possible, they try to look healthy when out in public. Kevin, for example, says, "Every time I go out [to a bar] I try to hide it. I try to act energetic and normal and I always have them put a squeeze of lime in my drinks so it's like a mixed drink." When their health makes it impossible to appear normal, they stay home. As David explains, "There are days that I really feel shitty and I look bad and I won't let anybody see me. I won't go around anybody. And then there are days I really force myself to put myself together so I will look decent and I'm not afraid to go out then."

This strategy is no help on days when individuals must go out despite visible symptoms. To protect their secret in these circumstances, individuals must devise plausible alternative explanations for their symptoms. In the early stages, they can claim that their weight loss is caused by stress or exercise, and that other symptoms are caused by minor illnesses, such as colds or the influenza. In the latter stages, they can claim that they have some other serious, but less stigmatized illness, such as leukemia or cancer.

Although hiding one's illness offers some protection against rejection, it carries a high price. Relationships with friends and families suffer when persons with HIV disease feel it is unsafe to discuss their illness with these others. At the same time, individuals forfeit any emotional or practical support they might otherwise receive from those who do not know of their illness. In addition, persons with HIV disease risk losing their jobs when they can offer no acceptable reason for their reduced productivity and increased absences. As a result, they eventually must disclose the nature of their illness to at least some individuals.

Following disclosure, individuals can avoid further stigma and emotional stress by reducing contact with those who prove unsupportive. As a result, however, their social lives shrink significantly. As Kevin says, "[Before getting ARC], I was out all the time. I loved to be around people. I hated to be by myself. But now, I find that I don't like to be around people that much except if it's people I know are not going to reject me because I don't want the rejection. I don't want to be hurt. I'm tired of being hurt."

To cope with losing their former social ties to friends, colleagues, and relatives, individuals can join support groups or participate in other social activities organized specifically for those who share their illness. In this way, they can garner the benefits of a social life without risking rejection or social awkwardness. Jeremy explains that he mostly socializes with others who have HIV disease "mainly because I guess I'm still afraid of people's reactions" but also "because I think they [those who have this illness] can understand more what your feelings are, what is going through your head. It's a lot easier to sit around and have a conversation with someone who is also ill with this disease, and you don't have to worry about avoiding certain topics." Persons with HIV disease also benefit from participating in these activities because everyone in these groups is stigmatized. As a result, the illness loses its "shock value" and instead becomes something that can be taken for granted. Consequently, they can engage in normal social interactions rather than interactions that are strained by the constant awareness of the illness. For example, Caleb, who was abandoned by most of his friends, tells of his pleasure at attending a potluck social for persons with HIV disease. At the potluck, he learned that he "was not alone":

I met a lot of really beautiful people, a lot of really nice friends. They took your phone number. They call you, socialize with you. You go to the show with them. You do things with them. If you need any help or whatever, they're there. . . . I went through hiding myself in my house and every time the facial sores started I would be afraid to go out and let people see me. These people don't care. You're not the only one that's had the facial sores and they don't care. You're welcome there. . . . Nobody [at the potluck] was afraid because a person with ARC or AIDS made a dish. We all rather enjoyed the food. It was like all the barriers went down when you were with these other people.

For those who live outside of the state's two major metropolitan areas, however, this strategy is unfeasible. It is also emotionally unfeasible for those who feel uncomfortable in groups that are solely or predominantly composed of gay men. Heterosexuals who do go to these meetings often conclude that they are wasting their time because the problems the groups discuss differ too greatly from their problems. Finding and informing new sexual partners, for example, is a difficult problem for all who have HIV disease. The particular issues involved, however, and the particular strategies one can use to cope differ for gay men and for heterosexuals, because the former but not the latter function in a sexual community in which everyone is presumed to be at risk for HIV disease and many already know that they are infected.

Even for gay men, support groups are mixed blessings. Although socializing with persons who have HIV disease solves some problems, it creates others. Because these persons often have only their illness in common, the relationships they develop with each other can be superficial and unrewarding. In addition, as Brent explains, these social circles do not permit him or other persons with HIV disease "to get away from AIDS and be myself at the same time." Only with others who have the same illness can they abandon the facades they use to protect themselves from social stigma.

Yet when they are with such others, they cannot avoid thinking about their illness. Moreover, those who become friends must cope with their friends' illnesses and dying as well as their own. As a result, the pleasure derived from support groups can turn to pain. Once this happens, individuals may decide to protect themselves emotionally by withdrawing from support groups and social networks made up of persons who share their illness.

Reducing Stigma

Although both hiding one's illness and restricting one's social circle can help persons with HIV disease avoid stigma, they will not reduce that stigma. Consequently, some individuals, like others who are stigmatized by society, consider these strategies inadequate and choose to attack the roots of that stigma directly.[2]

The decision to come out of the closet about their illness is not an easy one. Several men and women I interviewed would like to do so, but their doctors, husbands, friends, and relatives, fearing the potential for stress and stigma, have urged them not to. These warnings are particularly effective with those who have children and who fear that their children might also be stigmatized if their diagnosis becomes known.

Nevertheless, some do choose to reveal their condition publicly. They work for community organizations that deal with HIV disease, serve as "resources" for acquaintances who have unanswered questions about the illness, or even speak to the media about their situation. Those who take these actions believe that it is the only way to truly improve their situation. For example, after his friends shunned him and his mother refused to help him obtain health insurance, Hugh decided to speak out publicly about having ARC. He explains, "The only way that I could see getting rid of that stigma is to stick up for myself and become publicly known, to say it's okay to be my friend, it's okay to hug me, it's okay to sit down on a couch with me and watch TV." Other individuals continue to conceal their own diagnoses but nonetheless try to teach those around them that persons with HIV disease should not be shunned. David, for example, describes a confrontation with a neighbor who accused him of having AIDS and asked him not to use the pool in their apartment complex. David denied that he had AIDS, but also told the neighbor that "ignorance is no excuse. You ought to read up on AIDS—you can't get it that way."

To reduce stigma, individuals not only must educate others about the biology of their illness, but also must challenge the idea that it is a deserved punishment for sin. They do so in two ways. First, gay men who have HIV disease can argue that God is the source of love and not of punishment and that God would not have created gay people only to reject them as sinners. Second, all persons with HIV disease can argue that illnesses are biological phenomena and not signs of divine judgment. They also can assert that it was simply bad luck that the first Americans affected by HIV disease were gay men or drug users. Gay men who have HIV disease seem especially likely to argue that this illness originated with heterosexuals in Africa and thus cannot be a punishment for homosexuality. As Chris says, "It didn't start out as a homosexual disease and it's not going to finish that way."

These alternative explanations for their illnesses allow Chris and others like him to reject their rejecters as prejudiced or ignorant. Others, however, themselves believe that they deserve HIV disease. Such individuals can attempt to reduce stigma through what Goffman terms "apologies."[3] Instead of offering excuses for their behavior, these men and women first accept responsibility for their drug use or, more commonly, homosexuality and affirm their belief in the social norms that label those activities immoral. Second, they claim that they have reformed and are no longer the person who engaged in these activities. On this basis, they ask their families, churches, and God to accept their apologies, forgive their former sins, and believe that the new persons they have become are their real selves.

Finally, persons with HIV disease can reduce stigma through

bravado—putting on what amounts to a show to convince others of the reality of their situation, that they are, in fact, still functioning and worthwhile human beings. David describes how he and other persons with HIV disease occasionally go to a bar to "show these people that we can live with AIDS. That we can have a good time. That we can dance, that we can socialize, that we're not people with plagues." Describing a recent visit to a local bar, he says, "I just walked in, put my arms around somebody, said 'Hi, how're you doing? Everything going ok with you?' and he said, 'Well, how are you doing?' and I said, 'Well, ARC hasn't gotten me down yet. I don't think it will.' I said, 'I'm going to beat this thing.' And I just acted like nothing was wrong."

Living with HIV Disease

As their illness progresses, both the concerns of persons with HIV disease and the resources available to them shift. Stigma becomes a less critical issue, as their interactions with others necessarily become more limited and as they develop a supportive, if narrower, circle of friends, relatives, and health care workers. With time, too, the shock individuals feel at how some of their relatives and friends have reacted lessens, and they learn to accept the distance between them and those who once were close. Calvin, who was completely rejected by his family, says:

> Like anything else, any other disappointment that you have in life, you adjust. You categorize it in a fashion that's comfortable to you and you put it on the shelf with the rest of your hurts and you get on with your life. You don't let it destroy you. There's nothing wrong with hurting as long as you don't stay in that position too long and hurt for too long of a time. I can't change AIDS and I can't change my family, so I accept and go forward. That's all I can do.

Time also can help individuals recover from their own feelings of shame. At the follow-up interview, Brent, whose diagnosis had changed since the first interview from ARC to AIDS, said:

> In the beginning I had horrible feelings of dirtiness. Just the "leprosy" [feeling] was just overpowering. I wanted to hide it from the world. As I've had a time to accustom myself to having this and give myself time to think and rationalize and come to intellectual ideas rather than emotional responses, the feelings are less. . . . I've changed and become accustomed to it and I'm used to the idea.

As stigma recedes as an issue, and as the physical consequences of their illness become more overwhelming, other concerns come to the forefront. With the changes in their bodies, persons with HIV disease increasingly lose the ability to meet their own expectations for how they should perform in the roles and relationships that they retain. This loss of abilities and the resulting failed performances seriously threaten individuals' self-concepts. Psychologists have documented that, whenever possible, people will avoid recognizing any evidence that might force them to change their self-concepts, especially if that evidence might result in lowering their self-esteem.[4] The desire to maintain a consistent self-concept and level of self-esteem leads people to assume that their own motives are pure, acknowledge only favorable evaluations from others, recall and take credit for successes but not failures, and perceive new data selectively so as to confirm their preexisting self-concepts. Given the overwhelming changes produced by HIV disease, however, these strategies cannot work for long. As a result, as their illness progresses, individuals must develop ways to maintain their self-concepts and self-esteem despite unavoidable evidence that their lives have changed. To do so, they must construct new philosophical frameworks that allow them to downgrade the importance of their losses and to value the persons they now are and the lives they now lead.

To begin with, persons with HIV disease can reevaluate the importance of physical appearances. Typically, those I interviewed report that whereas previously they had thought "if I lose my looks I'll lose everything," now they believe that "the important thing is that I'm alive." As a result, they can separate their ideas about their appearance from their ideas about their inherent self-worth.

Similarly, persons with HIV disease can reevaluate their ideas about the importance of sexual activity; this is especially relevant for gay men. As those activities diminish, they may learn to value relationships that provide friendship more than those that provide sexual gratification. In addition, as their social circles shrink due to both stigma and their diminishing physical abilities, individuals quickly learn who are their true friends. As a result, they often feel that their remaining relationships with friends and lovers are now better and more meaningful than ever before. They therefore are able to replace their former self-concepts as sexual beings with new and equally valued self-concepts as loving beings.

Persons with HIV disease also find worth in their lives and their selves by emphasizing past accomplishments or present joys rather than future losses. This strategy additionally aids individuals by restoring some of their sense of control over their lives, for they can assert far more control over how they conceptualize the past and experience the present than over what will happen in the future.

Chris's case illustrates how one can derive a sense of self-worth by focusing on the past rather than the future. A former alcoholic now diagnosed with AIDS, Chris has made peace with the thought of his death by emphasizing what he has accomplished in his life. As he says, "I used to think about it all the time, that I didn't want to die. . . . But I'm proud of my life. I've changed it. I've done something with it. . . . I've stayed sober and I've passed along some sobriety to people. I've helped some people understand it, and that's important."

Other individuals deemphasize their diminished futures by stressing the benefits of focusing on the present and deriving pleasure from the wonders of everyday life. This is an especially important change for those whose previous focus on future goals had left them perennially dissatisfied with their lives. As a result, persons with HIV disease can experience greater happiness than ever before. Robert, who also has AIDS, says, "I think I just enjoy life so much more now. Everybody I come into contact with, it seems I notice the good things about them. You notice the flowers more. . . . You notice the sky more. You just notice all the things that are created in this world, and most all of them are beautiful. . . . I think I've gained life, actually [from having AIDS]. The beauty of it and what it really means, the caring, the sharing, the pretty flowers, the ugly flowers, the weeds or whatever, the sunshine, and the rain. I like all of it now."

Similarly, some individuals (especially those who used drugs) in the past had not taken their own lives very seriously. They had let things happen to them rather than trying to direct their fates. Now that they recognize that their life spans are short and finite, they are much more conscious about every choice they make—how they spend their time and with whom, what they eat and wear, how they interact with others, and the like. With this new consciousness, they can now choose how to live their remaining days so as to bring them happiness. As a result, HIV disease can seem more like a gift than a curse.

In sum, by changing their ideas about physical appearances, sexual activities, and the relative worth of past, present, and future, persons with HIV disease can limit the damage their illness can do to their self-esteem and more global self-concepts. Perhaps more surprisingly, they can develop new cognitive frameworks that enable them to use their illness not just to maintain but actually to improve their self-esteem. As individuals discover within themselves the emotional resources needed to confront illness, stigma, and dying with dignity, their self-esteem can increase. Similarly, as their experiences with HIV disease teach them a new compassion for and understanding of others, individuals can redefine themselves as less selfish and more humane than they had previously thought. Sarah, who now works for a community organization that deals with HIV disease and has begun organizing a support group for women, says, "I used to be a really stressed-out, rat-raced, job-oriented person, always put my careers ahead of my relationships. I'm just not like that [anymore]. I'm a much more caring person toward other people. I just take one day at a time. I relax. I've mellowed out and I'm a much better person for it." Clint derives similar benefits from helping others in his support group. He attends the group because he has, he says, "a very positive outlook on this thing [AIDS]. And if I can help those people that are having a very difficult time adjusting, and give them some of my energy, then I'm doing some good. I'm doing my part."

Political activism can also allow individuals to develop enhanced selves. This is especially true for those who can no longer contribute to the world through their work. David, who has appeared on the local news to describe his problems in obtaining social security benefits, recalls, "I didn't want everybody to know. But . . . once it was over and done with, I felt good about what I had done. Because it wasn't only for me that I was doing it. It was for a lot of other people out there that got the same problem." Similarly, others I interviewed point to their participation in this and other research studies as "legacies" that they are leaving to help others.[5] Calvin, explaining why he agreed to do the interview, says, "It's important to me to try to do something for mankind. To create enough interest that somebody will do something." Activities such as these help individuals to supplant failed performances in old roles with successful performances in valued new roles, and thus to maintain their self-esteem.

In addition, persons with HIV disease believe that they can help others simply because their deaths will add to the toll from this illness. They believe that, as that toll rises, the government eventually will have to devote more resources to seeking a cure or vaccine. Calvin continues, "I feel that I am making a positive approach toward mankind with dying from AIDS. . . . I feel that with my dying from AIDS I am becoming part of the statistics.

Once there is enough statistics, then somebody is going to do something about it, but they are not going to do anything until there is an emergency." This philosophy allows individuals both to find meaning in their suffering and to retain a sense of worth.

For gay men, having HIV disease can also improve their self-esteem by making them more comfortable with their sexuality.[6] Several report that in the past they had experienced considerable guilt and ambivalence about their lifestyles. Although they had engaged in gay sexual activities, they had found it difficult to embrace gay identities. Their illness has enabled them to integrate their sexual activities and sexual identities into coherent sexual self-concepts in one of two ways. For some, the process of dealing with a fatal, sexually transmitted disease has caused them to reexamine their feelings toward being gay. In this process, some have found a new self-acceptance. As Dick says, "I think I'm more comfortable with myself, now that I've had to deal with it [being gay] again. It's almost like coming out again. You can come out feeling better about yourself and feeling better about being gay." Having HIV disease also helps some men feel more comfortable with being gay by allowing them to see other gay men in a new and more favorable light. Tom has lived a very closeted life and has never had a serious relationship with another man. His feelings toward other gays have changed dramatically since becoming ill:

> The [gay] people I've seen caring for other persons with AIDS and so on made me realize that there can be a spiritual depth in the homosexual that I didn't realize there was before. My primary experience with homosexuals was in bars or bath houses and not a very positive experience. And to see people you might otherwise just have seen as being a hunk of meat or something like that actually caring for another person or going through all sorts of degradations in the disease process has really illuminated to me the fact that homosexuals are human beings.

In this way, their experiences with HIV disease enable some individuals who engage in gay activities to embrace gay identities for themselves.

For other gay men, HIV disease can eliminate dissonance between their sexual identities and sexual activities by ending those activities. Once concern about infecting others or worsening their own health forces them to abandon sexual activities, they no longer face contradictions between those activities and their sense of who they are or should be. Subsequently, both they and their families may stop considering them either deviant or sinful. As a result, they experience both more peace with themselves and improved self-esteem.

Dying with HIV Disease

As their health declines and death seems increasingly close and inevitable, persons with HIV disease must come to grips with the reality of their own mortality. To do so, they must once again develop a new set of cognitive frameworks which both makes their illness comprehensible to them and clarifies their options. Once they conclude that their illness will be fatal, they can make peace with their lack of control over their impending deaths by attempting to assert control over the nature of their dying.

Initially, HIV disease can seem an unfathomable mystery, which produces overwhelming uncertainties about its origins, nature, and consequences. Nevertheless, persons with HIV disease do develop explanations for why illness struck them specifically. In addition, over time, individuals develop ideas about the nature and consequences of HIV disease that enable them to understand and accept the changes in their bodies. Dick, for example, was diagnosed with ARC at the time of the initial interview and with AIDS at the time of the follow-up interview. He describes how he has come to terms with the uncertainty his illness has created:

I remember, a little over a year ago when I was first told what I had, it was very frightening. . . . You didn't know what the future held. A lot of that has been, at least, resolved. I don't worry about it so much as I did in that respect. It's still not something I want, but I guess you learn to live with it a little better. Then, when you get a case of pneumonia you know what it is, and you don't really think anything of it, other than the fact, that, well, "We know what's caused this."

In addition, as time passes, the uncertainty persons with HIV disease feel about the consequences of their illness not only is reduced but also becomes an accepted part of life. Stress decreases as individuals learn both to assert control over some aspects of their lives and to accept that they cannot control other aspects. For example, at the time of the first interview, David had ARC. By the followup interview, he had been told by his doctor that he was on the border of AIDS. Comparing his feelings at the initial and follow-up interviews, he says, "All I think I've done is adjust to it. I'm not so afraid. I guess I have realized that there's nothing that I can do about it."

Although most persons with HIV disease continue to hope for a cure, eventually their frenetic search for one abates, both because they lose hope and because they learn that the constant search for a cure can be physically and emotionally damaging. Jill, for example, describes how initially she would try to "do everything":

But you see what that means is I'd get real hyped [on] things in the newspaper, the media, you know, cures and stuff. . . . [But] I knew if I got that high I'd have to come down and get that low. Do you what I mean? So then I'd get real high about cures or ideas. Or I'd read something, you know, "This is wonderful!" And, you know, "This is going to just—this will do it. This will save my life." And, "This will make some of the things better." And then I'd get real high about that and

I'd rush around and get real positive. And believe it or not, it wasn't real healthy because, you know, I'd either be so physically exhausted from just being so hyper about something that the next day I'd either sleep all day or I would have a depression. It's the highs and lows that get you.

Jill no longer will read stories about HIV disease in the newspapers, but instead relies on her doctor to let her know of any new drug she should try.

Robert, who has AIDS, describes a different set of dangers persons with HIV disease can face if they start believing in a cure. He had taken zidovudine for a while, but was forced to stop because of life-threatening loss of blood cells. He says:

People with AIDS need to realize they are sick, deathly sick. I had got where I think you start feeling good which I guess it was because I was on AZT [zidovudine] too. It is the difference between black and white, night and day, or whatever. The first time I went on it I lasted six weeks. It was just marvelous. I just felt so good. Then the next time it didn't work for but a week and the next time it didn't work for but a week and I got scared. I had forgotten the possibility of dying.

This experience convinced Robert that he would be happier if he accepted his fate than if he continued on an emotional roller coaster of false hopes.

Those who conclude that nothing will cure them or restore their quality of life may decide to stop trying to preserve their lives. Calvin has stopped taking all medications:

At first, I got on the bandwagon of vitamins and getting nutrition and proper meals and eating my spinach and everything. One day I finally said: "What for?" It's not going to save me. I don't know of anybody that has not died from AIDS just because they ate spinach. . . . You can't run from AIDS. There's nowhere to go. If it's any other illness, then you have hope, you have dreams, you have treatment. With AIDS you don't. You just simply don't have an alternative to dying.

Calvin, like Robert, has decided that resigning himself to his fate is less distressing than trying to fight it. By so doing, he can now feel that he is once again making choices about what will happen to his life, albeit from a limited and perhaps self-destructive set of options.

Once persons with HIV disease decide that death is inevitable—and to some extent regardless of how sick they currently are—their conception of the future narrows. A striking feature of conversation with these men and women is the telescoping meaning of the future, as their long-range perspective shrinks and they move from talking about the future in terms of years from now, to months, weeks, or even hours. Sharon, for example, who has ARC, feels that her future has been "snatched away" from her. She says, "I don't feel the future exists for me any longer. [In the past] I would think about ten or twenty years down the road when I would be at a certain point in my life. Now I don't think about that. I think about each day."

In this narrowed future, death looms increasingly close. The regrets individuals feel center on the pain their death will bring to others and on their own loss of potential experiences, as they realize that they will miss seeing various future events, from their children's marriages to the price of strawberries next year. Jeremy, for example, says, "I regret that I probably will never make it to the point where I'll be one of those old men sitting in the malls drinking coffee, watching." A wistfulness, rather than bitterness, pervades most such remarks.

The meaning of death, however, is not overwhelmingly negative. For those who have firm Christian convictions, death can take on especially positive connotations of salvation and rejoining God in heaven. Religion can become a "fortress in the storm"—a source of strength in this world and hope about the next—especially if they find sympathetic clergy who will listen to their fears and sorrows and provide "unconditional love."

As their physical pain increases, death also can come to seem a blessing. Calvin emphatically states, "I'm so miserable now I pray to the Lord every night that he takes me. I cry myself to sleep just begging to die. I want to die so bad I can't hardly stand it. Not because I'm suicidal, but because I hurt. I hurt and I want it over with."

Although death can lose its power to frighten persons with HIV disease, however, dying retains its horror. Carol echoes the sentiments of most others when she says, "I'm not afraid to die. I may be afraid of the *way* it's going to happen, but I'm not afraid to die." Similarly, Dennis, who has already suffered one agonizingly debilitating episode, says, "Death doesn't bother me. Being ill as I was terrifies me." As these quotes suggest, the greatest fears of persons with HIV disease typically center on being kept alive against their will beyond the point where pain or disability makes their lives no longer worth living.

Such feelings led Dennis, along with several others I interviewed, to make plans to commit suicide should that seem warranted so that he could maintain his sense of control over the nature of his dying. As Dennis explains, "If I'm going to die, I would rather it be my business. I guess it's a lack of control. I want to reassert as much control as I can." Others have decided to let the disease take its natural course. They have signed living wills to prohibit physicians from keeping them alive through extraordinary means, instructed relatives not to let them be placed on life-support systems, and decided to stop taking their medications once life no longer seemed worthwhile. As Calvin, who has thrown away all his medications without informing his physician, explains, "I don't want to die, but I don't have a choice. I have to—period. I mean, no question. So if I have to die, why not tackle the chore and get it over with?"

Conclusions

For some individuals, having HIV disease can result in a "preoccupation with loss" that leaves them floundering in despair, unable to develop any strategies for coping with the impact of illness on their lives.[7] As this chapter demonstrates, however, many PWAs, like others who experience traumatic changes in their lives, can find ways to manage the changes in their social relationships, physical appearances, and physical abilities and to respond to the realities of a fatal illness.

This chapter offers significant additions to our understanding of how ill persons can manage stigma, their changing self-concepts, and their impending deaths.

The strategies persons with HIV disease use to avoid stigma (for example, hiding and selectively disclosing information) closely resemble those described by other scholars who have studied the experience of illness. The ways in which persons with HIV disease attempt to reduce stigma, however, have rarely if ever been documented. Gussow and Tracy previously have described how ill persons (specifically, those with leprosy) can become advocates for a social reappraisal of the meaning of their illness.[8] Neither they nor other researchers, however, have described how individuals can attempt to reduce stigma through apologies if they believe that stigma is justified. Nor have previous researchers described how ill persons or other stigmatized groups can, while circumventing the issue of whether stigma is justified, attempt to reduce stigma through bravado.

Similarly, other researchers (most notably, Kathy Charmaz) have documented the traumatic impact illness can have on individuals' self-concepts. Charmaz also has described how individuals can attempt to maintain self-esteem by either ignoring the changes in their bodies (striving for a "supernormal" or "restored" self) or focusing on the few remaining elements of their former selves (the "salvaged" self).[9] Although Charmaz alludes to the possibility that ill persons can find positive meaning in their illness, neither she nor other writers have explored how ill persons, like those described in this chapter, can develop enhanced selves through developing new values that allow them to define their current selves and lives as equal to or more valuable than their previous ones.

These coping strategies undoubtedly are also used by persons faced with other chronic and terminal illnesses. Certainly a major focus of many voluntary organizations, such as the American Diabetes Association and the Epilepsy Foundation, is to educate the public about these illnesses and to dispel the myths that lead the public to stigmatize affected individuals. And certainly many who have these illnesses, whether or not they belong to these organizations, also try in their personal lives to challenge the idea that they deserve either illness or stigma.

It is more difficult to see how the concept of "apologies" applies to other illnesses, for relatively few ill persons believe that they deserve to be stigmatized. For those who consider alcoholism an illness, however, the parallel is clear. One of the main (if perhaps unintended) purposes alcoholism treatment programs serve is to provide recovering alcoholics with believable "apologies," in which they both take responsibility for their past actions and request forgiveness on the basis that they have reformed.

Without question, bravado can be used by ill persons regardless of their illness. Bravado occurs whenever ill persons go beyond the introspective process of believing in the "restored" self that Charmaz describes and instead actively assert to others that their lives are essentially unchanged by their illness. Similarly, we can logically conclude that those who have other illnesses, given sufficient time, social, and emotional resources, can find sources of joy and pride in their lives and can devise ways to feel in control of their dying and to give meaning to their deaths.

CHAPTER 8

The Doctors' Perspectives

The effects of the HIV epidemic have rippled far beyond the lives of those who have this illness. One of the groups most directly affected has been doctors, who must decide whether and how to treat persons with this new, deadly, infectious, and stigmatized disease. Drawing on interviews I conducted with twenty-six Arizona doctors (as described in Appendix 2), this chapter examines the problems faced by doctors who treat persons with HIV disease.

The Decision to Treat

Except in very limited and specific circumstances, American doctors legally can refuse to provide care to new prospective patients.[1] Until 1988, the American Medical Association and the American Dental Association similarly held that doctors had no moral obligation to provide care. Currently, the official position of both associations is that doctors should not refuse to treat patients simply because they have HIV disease.[2] Neither association plans to enforce this, however.[3]

How common is refusal to treat persons with HIV disease? Only three published studies have looked at this question, with varied results. Atchison and her colleagues report that 56 percent

147

of a random sample of dentists and dental surgeons in Los Angeles will not treat persons with HIV disease.[4] Richardson and his colleagues found that 76 percent of gay primary practitioners and an equal percentage of heterosexual specialists in Los Angeles will not treat persons with HIV disease whom they diagnose.[5] Those who do treat such individuals do so primarily for reasons that would be less compelling for doctors practicing in areas where HIV disease is less common.[6] Gay primary practitioners need the fees they receive from persons with HIV disease and fear that if they refuse to treat these individuals they will alienate and perhaps lose their other gay patients. Heterosexual specialists fear that if they refuse to treat persons with HIV disease they will alienate the primary practitioners on whom they depend for referrals. In contrast, Link and his colleagues found substantial willingness to treat persons with HIV disease. They report that 75 percent of interns and residents at four New York City hospitals where HIV disease is common willingly treat these patients.[7] This sample may be unusual, however, in that doctors unwilling to treat such individuals will probably avoid placements at such hospitals.

Half the doctors I interviewed consider it morally acceptable for doctors to refuse to treat persons with HIV disease if they fear infection or feel they cannot provide good care because of their personal prejudices or lack of knowledge. The rest believe that doctors have an obligation to learn enough about the illness so that ignorance, prejudice, and fear will not affect their ability to treat those who have it.

When asked why they decided to treat persons with HIV disease, the doctors most commonly responded that infectious diseases or gay patients are their specialty (46 percent). In addition, 39 percent decided to treat persons with HIV disease because they consider it every physician's duty. Finally, 23 percent decided to treat these patients because of their commitment to serving the gay community. (These reasons were not mutually exclusive).

Despite these values, 21 percent sometimes think they "made

the wrong decision" in agreeing to treat persons with HIV disease. Such feelings were far more common among gay and bisexual doctors than among heterosexual doctors (57 percent versus 8 percent). Treating persons with HIV disease is especially difficult for gay and bisexual doctors for several reasons.[8] First, many of these patients are friends or long-standing patients, so the emotional costs of watching them deteriorate are high. Second, treating persons with HIV disease confronts these doctors with their own potential fate. Third, if one is an unmarried man, a primary practitioner, and over age thirty, treating persons with HIV disease in effect identifies oneself as gay; 71 percent of the gay and bisexual doctors but only 6 percent of the heterosexual doctors said that others sometimes assume they are gay because they treat persons with HIV disease. In part as a result, 42 percent of the gay and bisexual doctors but no heterosexual doctors believe that others have avoided or rejected them because of their work with persons who have HIV disease. Similarly, 29 percent of the gay and bisexual doctors report worsened relationships with friends, 28 percent with staff, and 42 percent with patients. None of the heterosexual doctors reports such problems. (Relationships with family and colleagues were not significantly affected.)

Fear of infection also contributes to doctors' qualms about treating persons with HIV disease. Link and his colleagues report that 48 percent of the residents they interviewed experience moderate or major concern about acquiring HIV disease from their patients and 40 percent believe that caring for persons with HIV disease has moderately or extremely increased their levels of stress.[9] Fifty-six percent of the doctors I interviewed had worried initially, and 42 percent still worry about getting HIV disease from their patients. These fears are not unreasonable, for 44 percent say they do not always protect themselves against infection, either because they lack the time, believe physical barriers such as gloves hinder their clinical judgment, or believe such barriers are rarely necessary.

Diagnosis and Its Aftermath

Such medical concerns are minor stresses compared to the ethical, psychological, and social problems attendant on treating persons with HIV disease. Problems can begin from the moment a person who might have HIV disease enters a doctor's office. Doctors who treat many persons with HIV disease soon learn to recognize the early signs of infection. They therefore face a tremendous dilemma whenever they suspect that individuals who have sought treatment for some minor ailment also unknowingly have HIV disease. For doctors who specialize in treating gay persons, this situation is not uncommon. Doctors then must decide whether to tell the patients what they suspect. If they do not tell, the patients cannot implement behaviors (such as improving their diet or taking drugs) that might safeguard their health. Yet if they do tell, the patients risk both psychological stress and social stigma. Such situations are enormously stressful for doctors. Jerry, for example, is a gay primary practitioner with one of the largest AIDS caseloads in the state. He says:

> People come in with a boo-boo or this or that or the other . . . and there are many times that I can see the first signs that something's going on. . . . It's terrible. It's one thing when someone comes into your office and they're four plus sick and they already have an idea that they might have AIDS and you make the diagnosis. But when somebody comes in with a boo-boo on their knee and you notice the purple spot on the side of their neck [that indicates Kaposi's sarcoma]! You know, they come in with a boo-boo on their knee where they fell last night and they go out with a terminal illness. That is a devastating thing to do. And I don't know how to handle that.

Moreover, because doctors schedule only enough time to treat the presenting complaint, they may have to counsel a patient regarding having an unexpected terminal illness in a ten-minute appointment. Alternatively, if they spend more time with this patient, all their other patients that day will have longer waits and shorter consultations.

Once either doctor or patient suspects HIV disease, the next question is whether to test for the virus. Twelve percent of the doctors view HIV tests no differently from other medical tests, provide no special counseling, and meet any requests for testing. The rest express considerable concern about the possible psychological and social consequences of the test, particularly because in Arizona doctors must report the names of all who test positive to the state health department. Mark is a heterosexual primary practitioner. He had moved to this country several years ago from a country with few civil liberties. Perhaps for this reason, he is one of the doctors who seem most cognizant of the potential ramifications of reporting:

> I think [reporting someone] could be really devastating. If that information gets into the wrong hands it can threaten the individual's relationships with family, friends, work, take away any opportunity he might have of getting any health or any other type of insurance ever again. I try to project myself into a situation like that and it's just mind-boggling how devastating it could be. It basically would threaten an individual's social standing. It would transform a person's whole status in his social world.

Because of these concerns, doctors may prefer to treat based on clinical indications rather than to run HIV tests. In fact, 29 percent of the doctors surveyed by McKusick and his colleagues in the years before new drugs made early diagnosis and treatment medically advantageous said that they "actively discourage their risk group patients" from being tested.[10] In the meantime, doctors can encourage patients to prepare themselves in various ways for the worst. Steve is a heterosexual infectious disease doctor who practices in a small Arizona city. He recalls his instructions to a man whom he suspected had HIV disease:

> "Look, I really don't want to ask you too many questions because you've got a good job. You can afford health insurance. I don't want to know too much right now. . . . I don't want to document anything in you. What I would encourage you to do is get some health insurance before we start doing any snooping because we may find that you're uninsurable. If I don't look and don't find anything, no one can accuse me of not having played fair."

The decision to test for HIV cannot be postponed indefinitely, however. Before running any tests, though, these doctors are careful to explain both the potential benefits and the potential consequences. Steve is especially concerned about the possible consequences of testing because he believes word travels fast in his small city. As a result, he says:

> I always do want people to know that they are . . . risking their insurability. They may be risking their jobs. They may be risking their personal relationships. . . . There's got to be some real benefit to it. You don't simply do it out of dumb, idle curiosity.

Those doctors who work for hospitals or clinics have their patients sign an informed consent form that delineates the potential legal, social, and psychological consequences of testing positive. In the past, to avoid the reporting requirements, some doctors encouraged patients to get tested out of state. Others suggested that patients use false names and in some cases arranged for them to do so. Interviewed before there were any places in the state that provided anonymous testing, Steve said:

> I really strongly, strongly, strongly encourage folks to get their tests drawn under an alias. What I do is send them

through from my office under an alias. I just hope there's no one by the same name. . . . But I always add a prefix. Like it's not Joe Blow but they go under Joe Blow the second, third, forth, fifth, sixth, seventh, eighth, ninth, tenth, eleventh. I think we're up to about sixteen or seventeen now.

If the results come back positive, the doctors' problems multiply, for they now must confront their conflicting obligations to their patients and to the state and the insurers. Marty, a gay primary practitioner with one of the highest numbers of patients with HIV disease says:

> Most patients . . . do not want any of this to be a part of their record because they won't be able to get insurance. The county will come after them and harass them. If their employer finds out it could be devastating to them. [So] . . . what do you do when an HIV patient comes to you? Do you put that in your record as you are supposed to and are required to do? Do you keep that part out of their record? It becomes very sticky. They want you to do this and then it's illegal to do that. You have to tell them, "Well, I can only go so far."

Some choose to ignore state law and keep the test results secret. Others feel they must report. Similarly, some do not report HIV test results to insurers. As Louis, a heterosexual infectious disease doctor who has treated many persons with HIV disease says, "Why should I tell the insurance company that this patient's HIV positive? Patients say 'I don't want them to know.' I don't feel any obligation that I need to, so I don't." Alternatively, doctors can circumvent legal requirements by reporting each opportunistic infection a patient develops but not identifying HIV disease as the underlying cause.

Few doctors are happy with this situation, or feel it solves their problems. Mike is a gay primary practitioner who treats many persons with HIV disease. He sometimes does not report HIV results. He says:

The social stigma of the disease leads to problems of record-keeping falsified. Oftentimes not fully putting down in the record everything that has gone wrong and reported in order to protect the patient's insurance [or] employment. And then trying to remember the next time I see them what I didn't write down. . . . It's a problem with me because I was taught to keep honest, complete, compulsive, medical records. And I find myself doing things that one side of me doesn't quite want to do.

Mark, who reports all cases, seems equally unhappy with his decision. Speaking of his first patient with HIV disease, he says:

It was very difficult for me to know what to do with the information when it became positive. I felt that it was really important for me to try to respect his request that this remain confidential. On the other hand, I knew that it was important, according to the legislation at the time, that all positives be reported to state health. I still have a difficult time knowing how confidential is confidential. The indications are rather threatening, not only in terms of breaching a trusting relationship with a patient but also the way I'd be setting myself up if I did not follow the rules and regulations with regard to my duties that I have to society in general.

Forty-two percent of the doctors believe that the need to protect confidentiality creates unusual legal risks for doctors who treat persons with HIV disease. These doctors cannot easily resolve the conflicts between their ethical values and their legal responsibilities.

Counseling Persons with HIV Disease

Because HIV disease is infectious, one of the first tasks a doctor faces following diagnosis is to counsel patients about how to protect others from infection. With the exception of those few infectious disease doctors who had once worked in venereal disease clinics and one or two others, this requires that they adopt a new and disconcerting role, for which they lack both training and experience, as sexual educators. The heterosexual doctors find it particularly uncomfortable to counsel the gay men who make up the bulk of their patients with HIV disease. Consequently, although none refuses to provide counseling about safe sexual activities, 85 percent only do so if asked directly.

Teaching patients how to use illegal drugs safely presents even greater difficulties for doctors, for this seems painfully inappropriate to many doctors. Almost half the doctors (46 percent) never teach how to clean needles. Those who do sometimes wonder if they are doing the right thing, for, as Jerry says, "It's a real tough place to put yourself in. Here you are as a healer and a physician and being antidrugs, telling somebody how to shoot up effectively." Their only alternative, however, is to tell patients to stop sharing needles or using drugs altogether—impractical advice, given that few drug users can get clean needles or get into drug treatment programs, and many have no interest in giving up drugs.

Even greater problems can emerge in subsequent weeks or months if the doctors learn that their patients either still engage in activities that can spread the virus or have not informed those they may have infected. In these circumstances, doctors face conflicts between their obligation to their patients and to those their patients may endanger. Reflecting legal precedents, the American Medical Association holds that in these circumstances, doctors should inform the authorities and, if necessary, the persons at risk.[11] Nevertheless, doctors faced with such situations may still agonize over how to proceed. As Mark explains:

> If someone does not want you to breach their confidentiality, it's rather difficult for me to deal with that, because I think it would be my responsibility to inform that individual's spouse if that person doesn't know. I think it's extremely im-

portant. I feel I'd be accountable if that person were to contract the disease and they knew that I had known about the
condition two or three years ago. They could probably have a
good cause to litigate. I also think that the person who has
the disease could litigate if I did not respect their rights. So
it's a rather difficult situation.

Treating Persons with HIV Disease

There is no cure for HIV disease. Nor is there any drug or combination of drugs that is guaranteed to keep the disease from progressing
(although zidovudine does seem able to slow its progression). As
a result, doctors receive frequent requests from patients who seek
potentially useful but illegal or experimental treatments.

The drug most in demand among persons with HIV disease is
zidovudine. Until recently, zidovudine was available only to those
few individuals who met researchers' requirements for experimental
subjects. This created serious ethical conflicts for doctors. To meet
the experimenters' criteria, Marty explains, "A lot of patients
wanted you to forge documents. It was something that at that time
I wanted to do for a lot of patients but I just could not do it, being
a professional. It's really tough when you see a patient who really
needs the medication and you cannot get it for him."

Other doctors had fewer qualms about bending the rules. To
circumvent the researchers' restrictions, a few doctors purposely
misdiagnosed patients so they met the criteria or gave away pills
researchers had allocated for deceased patients.

Zidovudine now is available by prescription to anyone with
HIV disease. Initially, however, the federal Food and Drug Administration (FDA) approved zidovudine for persons with full blown
AIDS but not for those at earlier stages of HIV disease. In response,
a few doctors continued to misdiagnose persons who did not meet
this criterion. Other doctors tried to obtain zidovudine legally by
petitioning the manufacturer for permission to prescribe it on a

"compassionate basis." The required paperwork was both time-consuming and aggravating, however. As Larry, a heterosexual infectious disease doctor who occasionally treats persons with HIV disease, says, "You don't get paid for that time. And that's extra time, and it's a lot of extra time. And it's not only extra time, it's time that isn't even fun or enjoyable. I don't mind talking with patients and not getting paid for it. But doing that kind of trash— yuck!" Moreover, there was no guarantee that the request would be granted. The doctors therefore had to weigh the benefits to their patients (and to their own finances) of spending their time providing direct services versus fighting the bureaucracy.

Although these problems no longer hold for obtaining zidovudine, they still apply for other experimental drugs. These difficulties pressure doctors to work outside the system. Marty, for example, helps others import promising drugs illegally because, as he says:

> I have become absolutely furious with what's going on with the bureaucracy in this country. I've gotten to the point where I've said, "I don't care, I'm going to do what I feel is right and if the bureaucracy comes after me I will pull out my sword and do battle with them as much as it takes." I have seen such stupidity, such heartlessness, such idiotic things occur that I have become very militant almost in my viewpoints about the bureaucracy.

Although only Marty admitted providing illegal drugs, 71 percent of the doctors interviewed will monitor the health of patients who use alternative drugs and 48 percent will refer them to persons who provide alternative drugs. For example, Jerry says:

> We do incorporate a lot of adjunctive non-FDA approved therapies. We don't necessarily direct those therapies but we will follow them. We don't necessarily prescribe them but we advise, "If you are going to use [the drug] DMCB as an immune

booster, this is the way that has been suggested to use it and these are the ways you need to be followed through blood tests. And these are the reactions you can expect and this is what you need to look out for. We will follow those on your routine visits. . . ." And for any of the other things that they may want to know about, I feel responsible that we be there to provide as much good information about those therapies as possible.

Providing Social Services

Doctors' efforts to obtain treatments for patients with HIV disease are seriously handicapped by the financial difficulties most of these patients experience. HIV disease almost invariably bankrupts its victims. Moreover, many persons with HIV disease lose the support of family and friends. As a result, many have no way to pay for medical care. Eventually, most become eligible for social security benefits and AHCCCS (Arizona's substitute for Medicaid). AHCCCS, however, typically pays only part of their subsequent bills from doctors who participate in that program. Thus, both before and after their patients get on AHCCCS, doctors must decide whether to provide care for which they may not be reimbursed. Those in private practice who have many patients with HIV disease report losing up to fourteen thousand dollars each year in unpaid bills.

The financial troubles of patients with HIV disease cost doctors time as well as money. The paperwork and telephone calls required by AHCCCS far exceed those required by other insurance plans. Moreover, many persons with HIV disease lack food, clothing, and shelter as well as medical coverage. Although some doctors avoid learning of these matters, others believe it is useless to provide medical care to patients who lack basic necessities. They therefore find themselves increasingly spending time negotiating with government bureaucrats and social service agencies to make practical arrangements for their patients. These additional time demands can create palpable resentment. As Mark explains:

> They [the persons with HIV disease] will call from an emergency room. The insurance carrier will call and want to know more about what's going on with this person. . . . A lot of these people are in insurance programs where as an entry to the health care system they have to go through my office. I'm what they call a primary care physician or gatekeeper. And for some of the logistics to happen, we have to make calls, and we have to participate in a way that we make the arrangements for these people. There's really nothing medical about it, but it takes up a great deal of time.

In addition, doctors may have to spend time counseling patients on their psychosocial problems, mediating between patients and their families, and serving as court witnesses in disputes between patients, their lovers, and their families. As Marty says:

> AIDS is an emotional disease as well as a physiological disease and I end up spending a lot of time refereeing battles between families and lovers. I just got through referring a battle over custodianship. A mother wanted to take her son away from his lover and her son didn't want to go and she went and got a court order. So you get involved in all of this kind of thing and then the court comes to you and wants you to give your opinion on who should have custody. . . . Then of course the mom is calling me and saying, "Well, you better tell them that I need that boy." And then the lover calls me, "Don't you dare let mom have this kid. He's perfectly fine, I can take care of him." So it's very tough. . . . I end up seeing a lot of nonmedical things and spending sometimes hours just talking to families and refereeing battles there.

Taken together, these additional time burdens lead 36 percent of the doctors to say that they sometimes resent the time they must spend on persons with HIV disease.

These time pressures are worsened by the need to serve as public educators. Because HIV disease is a new illness that has stimulated considerable popular debate and interest, doctors who are known to treat people with HIV disease are often called upon to answer questions about the illness from other patients, friends, reporters, and even other doctors. They may also receive frequent invitations to serve on various advisory boards and to lecture to hospital employees, local schools, and other community groups. The doctors can refuse some of these requests, but in other cases may feel morally or financially obliged to accept. Such obligations can significantly increase a doctor's workload.

When Death Nears

Because there is no cure for HIV disease, doctors who treat persons with this illness experience a significant increase in patient deaths. Before, even oncologists could anticipate that at least some of their patients would be cured or go into remission. The shift is particularly apparent to doctors in infectious disease, who have borne much of the brunt of the epidemic of HIV disease. For example, Barry completed his residency in infectious disease only a few years ago. He says:

> I was once told when I was interviewing for a fellowship by a famous old clinician that infectious disease is the only subspecialty where you really cure people. You don't cure people in cardiology and oncology. . . . And although infectious disease clinicians deal with very, very sick patients who often die— transplants, leukemics—we are not their primary physician so we don't usually have that onus, that weight, that, "Gee, if

we had just done something else things might have been better." Now we do.

Thus, doctors who treat persons with HIV disease must shift their focus from curing patients to simply alleviating their pain.[12]

Such a shift can bring considerable emotional turmoil. Several doctors expressed feelings of failure and guilt during the course of the interviews. Similarly, McKusick and his colleagues found that doctors who treat large numbers of persons with HIV disease report increased stress, fear of death, anxiety, and depression.[13] It is therefore not surprising that when asked what is the most difficult aspect of treating persons with this illness, half said simply and bluntly that their patients die.

As HIV disease progresses and death approaches, the main question doctors must grapple with is when to stop treatment. Doctors have a clear legal right to stop treatment if it is futile.[14] The problem, however, is in knowing when that point has been reached.[15] Moreover, doctors also may have to decide who should make that decision. Several factors make this issue more problematic in HIV disease compared to other terminal illnesses. Because patients with HIV disease are younger than most terminally ill patients, their lives may seem more worth extending. In addition, persons with HIV disease may want to have a lover (who lacks legal status) rather than a family member decide, or may have been abandoned by both lovers and family, leaving doctors with no clear guidelines regarding who should decide. Moreover, in the final stages, most persons with HIV disease become mentally incompetent and thus unable to make their wishes known and many deteriorate so rapidly that they can never make practical—let alone psychological—preparations for their death. Finally, because medical knowledge about HIV disease is growing so rapidly, 35 percent of the doctors and many patients believe that a cure will be found within the next five years—proportions that have probably increased since these interviews were conducted in 1988.

As Jonathan, an oncologist who has treated hundreds of persons with HIV disease, says:

> We know that with somebody who gets to a certain point in the cancer process, it is not reversible. And with AIDS I really do have the feeling that something special and miraculous is just around the corner. So that if you have somebody who is very debilitated but doesn't have complete degeneration of his brain, who knows that six months from now or three months from now something incredible will come along and we'll be able to reverse the process. We have no evidence, even for the dementia, that the manifestations of AIDS which kill the patients are irreversible, except [if] they have a widespread lymphoma or squamous cancer or something like that.

Thus it may seem worthwhile to keep an individual alive as long as possible.

All these factors make it difficult for doctors to decide when to terminate care and lead 75 percent of the doctors to conclude that it is more difficult to treat persons with HIV disease than to treat other terminally ill patients. This situation can be tremendously stressful for doctors, who are trained to heal but faced with an ugly death. Steve, for example, describing a patient he had treated for some time, says:

> He would have seizures. He would have gastrointestinal bleeds where he would literally fill the bed with blood passed per rectum. He became paraplegic. He had ongoing fevers to 103. He was a skeleton. I just kept thinking that this is so unfair that he doesn't die. This isn't fair to anybody. It's not fair to him. It's not fair to his parents. . . . I found myself just wishing that he could die. It was more awful than the worst nightmare that I can imagine.

Nevertheless, he kept providing treatment:

> And I finally said, "Isn't it sick that you want this fellow to die and here you are taking care of him?"

Since then, he has learned not to pursue such heroic measures:

> In AIDS, once a patient crosses a certain threshold, once their illness has progressed to a certain point, they have multiple problems, they have multiple infections. Everything is wrong, nothing works right. To pursue everything would be barbaric. The thing that's important is to keep the patient comfortable.

To reduce some of their burdens, doctors can discuss these issues with patients while the patients are still competent, and can encourage patients to get durable powers of attorney.[16] As Jerry notes, however, "These things are death-planning things, and that takes away from the positive approach that we want to take." Moreover, it may not be possible to do so, for patients may procrastinate or may already be mentally incompetent before one assumes care.

Conclusions

The central impact on doctors of treating persons with HIV disease stems from the changes in their role. Because of the unusual nature of HIV disease, treating such individuals means accepting new or expanded roles as negotiators with bureaucrats, sexual counselors, mediators with families, psychotherapists, and public educators. Most critically, it means shifting from healing to providing largely palliative care. In addition, when their ethical values and legal roles conflict, it requires many doctors to work outside or on the margins of the system for the first time.

Despite these changing roles, in many ways the impact on doctors who treat persons with HIV disease is limited. These doctors confront new problems but can integrate many of them into preexisting contexts. All doctors must occasionally give patients bad news, balance conflicting obligations, or make decisions about when to stop treatment. Although the particular factors involved in HIV disease make these situations more difficult for doctors, they already have a repertoire of medical and psychological skills that help them cope.

Thus, despite the problems that treating persons with HIV disease has caused for them, 73 percent of the doctors feel that they also have benefited in some way from treating these patients. The majority (71 percent) of the gay and bisexual doctors believe that their self-images have improved because it has helped them to embrace their own sexual identities, as they have been forced to confront more openly both their own homosexuality and others' homophobia. All the doctors have developed new medical skills and knowledge. And finally, 58 percent report that their experiences with persons with HIV disease have helped them to grow as persons. Jerry, for example, describing his interactions with such patients, says:

> I think it's a privilege [to treat these persons]. I'm very lucky in very many ways. I'm allowed to see into the lives of not only PWAs but their families in ways they would never show even other family members. It's a real privilege to have that kind of an intimacy. . . . And I see strength that comes from people who don't need to be strong. I see a real spiritual health in people who should be angry. I see forgiveness. . . . I see these wonderful positive things from people who are giving rather than taking those positive things at a time of need.

Such interactions can teach doctors a new appreciation for the wonders of life and a new respect for those less fortunate than themselves.

CHAPTER 9

The Future of HIV

HIV disease was first identified in 1981. By 1991, it will be one of the top ten causes of death in the United States and by far the most common cause of death for persons ages twenty-five to forty-four. Already, although cancer and heart disease cause far more deaths than HIV disease, the latter costs the country more years of lost economic productivity, because it affects a far younger population. Moreover, the number of new cases of HIV disease each year will continue to grow for many years, as more people become infected with HIV and as many of the millions worldwide who are already infected progress to full-blown AIDS.

The Prospects for a Vaccine

Because of scientists' limited knowledge about HIV, the difficulties of researching HIV, and the nature of HIV, the prospects for a vaccine to stop its spread are not good.

A central problem scientists face in developing a vaccine is their limited knowledge about retroviruses, the subset of viruses to which HIV belongs. Until the last few years, retroviruses were believed to attack only animals and to present only a minor threat even to those species. Scientists discovered that retroviruses

can affect humans only shortly before HIV disease was first identified. As a result, researchers have relatively little knowledge of retroviruses to draw on in developing treatments or vaccines.

Developing knowledge about HIV presents special difficulties
because scientists lack a useful animal model for this virus. The
only animals other than humans that can be infected with HIV-1,
the form of HIV that causes AIDS in humans, are chimpanzees.
Unfortunately, chimpanzees are too rare and expensive to use in
extensive research studies. In addition, although chimpanzees can
become infected with HIV-1 and develop some symptoms of HIV
disease, they do not actually develop AIDS. As a result, it is difficult for scientists to test vaccines on chimpanzees. Recently, however, scientists have learned that macaque monkeys do not respond
to HIV-1 but do develop AIDS following infection with HIV-2,
another form of the virus. Scientists do not yet understand how
HIV-2 differs from HIV-1. Nevertheless, this discovery lends hope
that the cheaper and more available macaque monkeys can be used
in researching vaccines.

What we do know about HIV suggests that it will be especially difficult to design an effective vaccine against it. Vaccines work
by infecting individuals with a safe variant of a disease-causing
virus. Once infected, the individual's immune system produces antibodies that recognize and destroy the virus should it subsequently
enter the body. For several reasons, the development of a vaccine
in this century is unlikely.[1]

First, HIV mutates more rapidly than most viruses. Many
different strains of HIV already exist. A vaccine that works
against one strain generally will not work against another strain.
This is why a vaccine against the common cold, for example,
which also has many different strains, is not feasible. An effective
vaccine would somehow have to work against all the different existing and future strains of the virus—a difficult, if not impossible,
task.

Second, scientists lack any natural model for a vaccine against
HIV disease. The search for vaccines against other diseases was

aided immeasurably by the existence of naturally occurring antibodies that prevented those diseases. Persons who had cowpox, for example, were protected against smallpox, and persons who survive one attack of measles are protected against future attacks. Scientists used their knowledge of how these antibodies work to develop vaccines against these diseases. Currently, however, scientists know of no such protective antibodies to HIV.

Third, the immune system protects individuals from disease by recognizing and attacking any foreign substances in the body. HIV, however, can remain hidden inside a cell without appearing in any form on the cell's surface. As a result, the immune system, even if somehow stimulated by a vaccine, will not know that a cell is infected and therefore cannot respond to that infection.

Fourth, even if scientists should develop a promising vaccine, they may be unable to conduct the necessary human tests. Volunteers would have to be informed that the vaccine might itself cause health problems. They would also have to be informed that, following injection with the vaccine, they would always in future test HIV-positive. Consequently, they would risk all the social and psychological burdens of that status with no guarantee that they were protected against HIV disease. If volunteers could still be found, scientists would have to devise accurate means of monitoring all drug use and sexual activity through which volunteers might become infected in order to ascertain whether the vaccine had protected them. This would create practical problems for researchers and the potential for stigma among volunteers. Alternatively, to test whether the vaccine worked, volunteers would have to agree either to engage in risky behaviors or to be injected with live virus. The inherent ethical problems and the potential for liability suits have dampened drug companies' and nonprofit agencies' interest in sponsoring such research, making it difficult for scientists to obtain the necessary funding. Finally, even if these problems could be solved, the long latency period between exposure to HIV and the development of symptoms means that scientists would not know if the vaccine had worked until several years had passed.

The Shifting Demography of HIV Disease

At least for the near future, therefore, the number of persons with HIV disease will continue to grow. With this growth will come important changes in the distribution of the disease, as it continues to spread inward from the two coasts and as it increasingly strikes drug users, heterosexual men and women, and children.

The geographic distribution of HIV disease has been shifting steadily for some time. Prior to 1983, 63 percent of all reported persons with AIDS lived in the mid-Atlantic states of New York, New Jersey, and Pennsylvania.[2] By 1988, the proportion had decreased to 32 percent, as cases of AIDS appeared across the nation. Nebraska, for example, had reported a total of 20 cases by the end of 1986 and a total of 127 by the end of 1989—a sixfold increase in only three years.[3]

The characteristics of persons who contract HIV disease are also changing. During the 1980s, most persons with HIV disease in the United States were white men. The majority were infected through homosexual intercourse. Sharing intravenous needles and heterosexual intercourse, the next most common sources of HIV infection, caused far fewer persons to become infected. As the population of gay men reaches its saturation point for HIV infection and as those who remain uninfected adopt safer sexual practices, fewer gay men will become infected each year. Drug use and heterosexual intercourse, meanwhile, are playing increasingly large roles in the transmission of HIV. For example, drug users have always comprised a significant proportion of AIDS cases in New York City. Only since 1988, however, has needle sharing caused the majority of the city's AIDS cases.[4]

The growing importance of drug use in the transmission of HIV in turn is putting more racial minorities, poor persons, women, and children at risk. Since it was first identified, blacks and Hispanics have been more likely than whites to contract HIV disease; nonwhites make up 20 percent of the U.S. population but have consistently comprised about 40 percent of U.S. AIDS cases.

Because intravenous drug use is more common in minority than in white communities, as drug use becomes a more important source of HIV transmission, minorities will become a larger proportion of all persons with HIV disease.[5] For the same reason, HIV disease is becoming a disease of the poor. This will be a significant change, for the early cases in the United States were disproportionately from the middle and upper classes; 53 percent of persons who died from AIDS in 1986, for example, compared to 37 percent of all U.S. adults, had attended college.[6]

Heterosexual transmission is also becoming a more important element in this country's HIV epidemic. Since the start of the epidemic, most persons with HIV disease in West Africa, where the rate of HIV disease is the highest in the world, have become infected through heterosexual intercourse. In the United States, however, relatively few individuals have become infected in this way. Most of those few were infected by sexual intercourse with intravenous drug users, rather than with bisexual men. As more drug users become infected, therefore, so will more of their heterosexual partners. Although few observers now expect the explosion of cases among heterosexuals that some once predicted, persons infected through heterosexual intercourse already are the fastest-growing group of adult AIDS cases in the United States.[7]

Not surprisingly, so long as most persons with HIV disease were infected through male homosexual intercourse, few women contracted HIV disease. With the increasing role of heterosexual intercourse in the spread of HIV, however, more women are becoming infected.

As more women become infected with HIV, more children will as well, for HIV can be transmitted from mother to fetus before birth and from mother to baby during birth or through breast milk. Pediatric HIV disease is already becoming more common, even though children with hemophilia (formerly the majority of pediatric cases) no longer risk infection now that blood is routinely tested for HIV before it is used in transfusions. The number of children with HIV disease will grow even more rapidly if current trends toward restricting access to abortion continue. Women with HIV disease are overwhelmingly poor at the time they become infected and usually become even poorer as a result of their illness. Most can obtain abortions only if they are available free through publicly funded facilities in their own communities, for few can afford to pay for abortions or to travel to other communities to obtain free abortions. Consequently, if the government further reduces public funding for abortion or legal access to abortion, many more women will be forced to carry pregnancies to term. Twenty to 50 percent of these babies will be born infected with HIV.

Not only will the future bring changes in who develops HIV disease, but it will also bring significant changes in when individuals learn that they are infected. To date, most individuals have learned this only after they started developing symptoms of some opportunistic infection, long after they were initially infected. Increasingly, however, individuals are learning that they are infected at far earlier stages.

The shift toward earlier detection of HIV disease is a result of both mandatory testing and routine, but voluntary, testing. Although most public health authorities believe that the social and economic costs of large-scale testing programs far outweigh the potential benefits, the U.S. government now tests all new military recruits, active duty military personnel, ROTC students, Job Corps and Peace Corps applicants, federal prisoners in all fifty states, prospective immigrants, and members of the Foreign Service and their dependents before any overseas posting.[8] In addition, some states now require HIV tests for all state prisoners, and others are considering such legislation.

Testing is now becoming routine, although still voluntary, in a variety of situations. Many hospital patients, pregnant women, persons who seek care at clinics treating sexually transmitted diseases, and others are now either routinely asked if they want to be tested for HIV or tested without their knowledge.[9] Thus, more and more persons are learning that they are infected with HIV before they develop any obvious health problems.

The Changing Nature of Life with HIV Disease

In sum, HIV disease will continue to spread across the nation in future years. Fewer persons with HIV disease will be middle class, white, or gay, and more will learn that they are infected with HIV early in the course of their illness. These geographic, demographic, and technological shifts will combine with shifts in the number and nature of health care workers who will treat persons with HIV disease to change the experience of living with this illness.

The Consequences of Earlier Diagnosis

Of these shifts, the one that seems most likely to benefit persons with HIV disease is the shift toward earlier diagnosis. A natural consequence of early diagnosis is that individuals will seek care earlier in the course of the illness. That care will consist of routine outpatient checkups to detect any health problems and of drug therapies to treat those problems. Early diagnosis can thus help individuals keep their health from deteriorating.

Unfortunately, few persons with HIV disease will have sufficient insurance coverage to pay for care in the early stages of the illness. As described, many lack any insurance coverage or will lose their insurance along with their jobs because of discrimination or ill health. The rest will soon learn that insurance companies less often pay for outpatient than for inpatient care, less often pay for drugs than for other forms of care, and less often pay for experimental drugs (a category that will continue to include many of the most promising treatments for HIV disease) than for established drugs.[10] Consequently, to pay for their care, many individuals will be driven into poverty while still in the early stages of the illness. Moreover, the burdens on the public health care system will expand significantly once these poverty-stricken individuals are forced to seek care from within that system. Arno and his colleagues estimate that if, in 1988, even 25 percent of persons infected with HIV but not yet diagnosed had sought prophylactic treatment, it would have cost more than $2.5 billion.[11] A large proportion of these costs would have been borne by the public health care system, further overburdening that system and further reducing the quality of care available to all patients, including those with HIV disease.

The psychological and social consequences of early HIV testing will be equally devastating. Because these tests are not foolproof and are especially likely to produce errors in low-risk populations, any broad extension of testing will swell the number of persons told that their serostatus is indeterminate or falsely identified as HIV-positive. Even if subsequent tests prove that they are uninfected, the psychological trauma of dealing with a false-positive or indeterminate test result will have been enormous. Moreover, some will have trouble ever believing that they are uninfected. In addition, even after tests prove that they are uninfected, some will find that their friends, relatives, employers, or others doubt this news and continue to stigmatize them. In addition, those who learn that they *are* infected will begin experiencing stigma far earlier than if they had been diagnosed only after symptoms appeared.

The one factor mitigating the effects of this stigma is the growing legal protection available to those who have HIV disease.[12] Since the early 1970s, state and federal antidiscrimination statutes have offered increasing protection to all disabled persons. Several recent court decisions have declared that these statutes apply to persons who have HIV disease. In addition, several states have passed new statutes specifically applying antidiscrimination principles to persons with HIV disease, and a federal statute to this effect is under consideration. Several states also have enacted laws to protect the confidentiality of HIV test results. As testing becomes more widespread and its social dangers more apparent, other states may do the same.

The Consequences of Geographic Changes

With the geographic dispersion of HIV disease, some problems that occurred in earlier years in the areas where the disease first struck will recur in similar form elsewhere. Persons with HIV disease living outside the cities where HIV disease is most common always have found it difficult to obtain an accurate diagnosis, get experimental drugs, or find support groups. These problems will continue as such individuals seek care in regions where their illness is still rare and where medical and support services are still underdeveloped. The quality of care available to them will also be lower in areas where health care personnel have limited experience with this illness; results from one small study suggest that persons with HIV disease are more likely to die if they are treated in hospitals where their illness is relatively rare.[13]

The social status of persons with HIV disease will also be worse in areas where this illness is just beginning to have an impact. By now, in places like New York and San Francisco, where HIV disease has been widespread for some time, many employers have developed policies for dealing with HIV-infected workers or clients. Their staffs, meanwhile, have become accustomed to working with those who have this illness. Far fewer employers and employees in other parts of the country have this experience and have made the necessary adjustments. Persons with HIV disease in the latter areas, therefore, will encounter discriminatory treatment like that faced by others in large coastal cities several years earlier. Moreover, those who attempt to fight this treatment will have to do so in areas (like Arizona) that are far more conservative politically and religiously than those in which the illness is now most common.

The Consequences of Demographic Changes

The lives of persons with HIV disease will change most significantly because of the spiraling proportion who must rely on the public health care system. Many persons with HIV disease are poor before becoming ill, and many more are bankrupted by their illness. For example, 66 percent of persons with HIV disease who died in 1986 compared to 39 percent of those who died from all other causes had less than five thousand dollars in assets at the time of their deaths, even though the former were two and one-half times more likely to have held managerial or professional positions before their illness.[14] Consequently, many persons with HIV disease cannot afford to pay for the treatment they need, for, unlike every other developed nation other than South Africa, the United States does not provide universal health coverage. Thus, they must either do without needed care or, if they can, rely on the public health system. Currently, 40 percent of persons with HIV disease pay for their care through Medicaid, and another 20 percent have no medical coverage.[15] These numbers will rise as the illness increasingly becomes an illness of the poor, who have neither insurance nor the cash to pay for their care.

Moreover, if current trends in insurance continue, more middle- and upper-class persons with HIV disease will also have to rely on the public health care system. In the last few years, private insurance companies have refined ways of limiting their losses due to HIV disease.[16] Some insurance companies now require negative HIV tests before they will issue individual insurance policies. Such requirements are legal except in the few jurisdictions, such as the District of Columbia and California, that have passed laws forbidding this practice. Others will not insure any men who are single or who live in areas where HIV disease is common. Still others will not insure men who work in stereotypically feminine jobs or who in other ways fit the insurers' stereotypes of gay men. In addition, some insurers specifically limit the benefits they will pay for HIV disease. Others will pay benefits to persons with this illness only if they can prove that they were uninfected when they obtained the insurance and that HIV disease was thus not a preexisting condition. Given the long latency period between initial infection and the development of symptoms, the only individuals who can do so are the few infected by an identified contaminated blood transfusion and the few who for some reason were tested for HIV shortly before obtaining insurance. Thus, even if more laws outlawing blatant discrimination in insurance are passed, more and more persons with HIV disease will find themselves either without insurance or with insurance that proves useless once they become ill. Consequently, they will have no choice but to turn to the public sector for their care.

To protect the public health system from bankruptcy, several states have established insurance risk pools. These pools insure individuals who are otherwise uninsurable and who by definition are bad risks. By pooling the risks of these individuals, states can keep the rates lower than they would otherwise be. Nevertheless, their premiums, copayments, and deductibles are still much higher than those most people pay for their insurance, and prohibitively high for some. Even with these higher rates, all but one pool lost money in 1986 (the last year for which figures are available).[17] To keep them solvent, the states provide partial subsidies from the state premium taxes that private insurance companies pay. Increasingly, however, employers are shifting to using self-insurance plans, which are untaxed; these plans now cover between 50 and 60 percent of insured workers.[18] Consequently, the subsidy available to state risk pools is shrinking, and these pools may soon become economically unfeasible.

Thus, in the future, many more persons with HIV disease will lack either private or publicly subsidized insurance and will be forced to turn to the public health care system. Yet this system is already becoming overwhelmed and the quality of care it can provide already is falling in the areas where HIV disease is most common. Although caring for patients with HIV disease costs no more on average than caring for other medical or surgical patients, revenues have not kept up with costs. In 1987, for example, hospitals lost an average of $136 per day for every AIDS patient they treated, compared to $26 per day for other patients.[19] Moreover, this burden is not distributed equally. Fewer than 5 percent of the nation's hospitals treat more than 50 percent of all persons with HIV disease. Those hospitals now risk financial ruin as a result of unpaid bills, as do other hospitals that have few patients with HIV disease but many who lack medical insurance; hospitals both in the Northeast, where HIV disease is relatively common, and in the South, where it is rare, but where the states provide medical insurance to only the most indigent, lost an average of $600,000 in 1987.

As HIV disease becomes more common among drug users and

women, hospitals' financial hardships are growing. For unknown reasons, drug users generally develop different opportunistic infections than gay men. Because the particular infections common among drug users cost more to treat than those common among gay men, the growing number of drug users with HIV disease will add to the financial burdens of hospitals and public clinics. In addition, drug users often are in poor health even before contracting HIV disease. Moreover, drug users more often than others with HIV disease lack homes or families to which they can be transferred if they require less intensive care. Consequently, many remain in hospitals longer than necessary.[20] As more drug users develop HIV disease, therefore, the financial burdens on hospitals will grow, and the quality of care they can provide will fall.

The growing number of women with HIV disease will also strain the health care system and threaten the quality of care it can provide. On average, women are poorer than men; in 1987, the median income for U.S. women was $8,101, whereas it was $17,752 for men.[21] Thus, even though women and men are equally often covered by insurance, women are less able to pay for drugs or services that their insurance does not cover and are more likely to leave unpaid bills in their wake. Moreover, women more often than men are abandoned by their husbands or lovers once they become ill. Consequently, as women become a greater proportion of persons with HIV disease, the proportion of patients who remain in hospitals simply because they lack homes will increase.

The one sign of hope for the public health care system has come from the city of San Francisco, which has managed to provide quality health care to persons with HIV disease despite extremely high rates of this illness. Between December 1988 and November 1989, the San Francisco metropolitan area reported 107.9 new cases of AIDS per 100,000 persons, almost twice the rate of the next-hardest-hit area.[22] Yet the cost of treating the illness is lower in San Francisco than anywhere else in the United States, even though the services provided are probably the best.[23] As a result, some observers have suggested that San Francisco can serve as a model for cost-effective, humane, and medically appropriate care for persons with HIV disease.

This model is not likely to work in other cities, however.[24] San Francisco has limited the costs of treating HIV disease by emphasizing outpatient rather than inpatient care. In contrast, the U.S. health care system in general favors inpatient over outpatient care, even though the former is more expensive. For example, health insurance plans are far more likely to pay for life-support systems for a hospital patient in a permanent vegetative state than to pay a fraction of that cost to provide the nursing and housekeeping care needed to allow individuals to die with dignity in hospices or their own homes. The city of San Francisco has attempted to switch these priorities. To do so, it has relied heavily on volunteers who provide hospice care, long-term home-based care, and the sort of daily household assistance (doing laundry, getting groceries, and the like) that allows persons with HIV disease to continue living in the community rather than in institutions.

This system has worked in San Francisco for two reasons. First, the city has heavily supplemented the meager federal funding received by the nonprofit agencies that provide these services. Second, these agencies have drawn on a preexisting, organized, gay community willing to provide services to those it considers its "own." For these same two reasons, this model is unlikely to work elsewhere. To date, other cities have proven far less willing than San Francisco to provide financial assistance to community organizations that deal with HIV disease. Recent increases in caseloads without increases in funding already have caused budget problems for many community organizations and forced them to cut back on their services to persons with HIV disease.[25] In addition, as drug users and their sexual partners replace gay men as the typical persons with HIV disease, both in San Francisco and elsewhere, the pool of volunteers will shrink, for no similar bonds unite these populations. Moreover, even in places where gay men remain the majority of persons with HIV disease, this model will not work forever. Even the most dedicated volunteers eventually burn out as the epidemic continues and people continue to fall ill. Consequently, the quality of care available to persons with HIV disease will decline, both in San Francisco and elsewhere, as the public health care system deteriorates and as the San Francisco model proves unfeasible.

Problems in Finding Health Care Providers

Even if the economic burdens of providing care to persons with HIV disease do not overwhelm the system, the quality of care they receive may still decline. Since the epidemic began, those who have this illness have encountered difficulties in finding health care workers willing to provide care. These problems may multiply in the future.[26] Anecdotal evidence suggests that some medical students are choosing specialties other than internal medicine and infectious disease to avoid working with persons who have HIV disease.[27] Similarly, some graduating medical students are seeking residencies in cities where HIV disease is rare because they fear becoming infected, abhor homosexuals or drug users, or worry that they will not get the well-rounded education they need if they spend too much time working with those who have HIV disease.

The same logic may lead other individuals to leave or decide against entering ancillary health care fields such as nursing, medical technology, and dental hygiene. In the past, these traditionally female fields, which offered low pay, hard work, and great stress, could recruit sufficient workers because women had few alternative sources of employment. As women's career options have expanded, the supply of workers in these fields has decreased significantly. The potential for infection with HIV has made these fields seem even less attractive. Moreover, because the demand in these fields far outstrips the supply, those who choose to enter them will have greater bargaining power and control over where they work. Some may exercise this control by avoiding practicing in settings where HIV disease is common.

In addition, some doctors and other health care workers who treated persons with HIV disease during the first decade of the epidemic are withdrawing from the field. Many entered this field because they themselves are gay and therefore felt a sense of connection with and obligation to other gays. As the proportion of gay men among persons with HIV disease declines, so will the sense of obligation felt by these health care workers. Any remaining feelings of responsibility to those who have this illness will be outweighed for some by the desire to avoid the psychological stress and, for those in private practice, the financial sacrifice of treating these persons.

As the population of persons with HIV disease shifts from educated, involved, and generally compliant gay men to poor and poorly educated drug users—a population notorious for its tendency to manipulate others and its limited compliance with medical regimens—the interest of heterosexual health care workers in treating persons with HIV disease will also decline. Moreover, observers often have noted that many doctors and nurses dislike caring for persons who have attempted suicide, believing that such persons do not deserve assistance.[28] Faced with difficult-to-treat patients who became infected because they chose to inject drugs, some workers undoubtedly will decide that these individuals chose their fate and do not deserve their help.

It is more difficult to predict whether the perceived risk of HIV infection will increase among health care workers and whether this, too, will lead some to avoid working with those who have HIV disease. As of February 1989, and even though needle-stick injuries are fairly common, the CDC had documented only thirteen cases of U.S. health care workers who have become infected with HIV through their work.[29] There is no reason for the *proportion* of exposed workers who become infected to increase. However, as more persons with HIV disease enter the system, and even if workers become more conscientious about protecting themselves against accidental blood exposure, the *number* of health care workers exposed to infected blood and the number infected through their work will rise. As a result, more and more health care workers will know, or know of, someone infected through their work. This will make the risk of HIV infection more salient and the desire to avoid working with those who are infected more compelling.

Other factors, on the other hand, will decrease the salience of this risk. For those who begin health care training in the 1990s, HIV disease will be a part of medical life. Like health care workers who trained prior to the 1940s, they will know that these fields entail certain risks. Before the development of antibiotics, for example, doctors and nurses accepted that tuberculosis was a common and often fatal occupational hazard. In contrast, health care workers who trained from the 1940s through the 1970s entered their professions expecting few personal risks. It is this generation that has been so surprised by and unprepared for the epidemic of HIV disease. The potential for HIV infection may seem considerably less overwhelming and unacceptable to those who train in future decades.

In addition, those who train in the future will learn from the start both how to treat persons with HIV disease and how to protect themselves from infection. Unlike older practitioners, who must change ingrained habits to protect themselves from infection, those who train in the future will be drilled in how to protect themselves. Similarly, whereas older practitioners must make special efforts to learn how to treat persons with HIV disease, those who train in the future will learn how to do so from the beginning. Consequently, future generations of health care workers will feel more competent at, and hence more comfortable with, treating persons who have HIV disease. Whether these factors will counterbalance the forces pushing individuals to avoid working with those who have this illness remains to be seen.

The Changing Social Construction of HIV Disease

Future years will also bring changes in the meanings attributed to HIV disease. Since it was first identified, the social construction of

HIV disease has made it an exceptionally stigmatized illness. This has happened because HIV disease is infectious, linked to sexuality, and associated with already stigmatized groups; causes disfiguring and dehumanizing changes, extensive disability, and death; threatens the social and economic fabric of society; seems mysterious; and cannot be prevented by a vaccine.

So long as these facts remain, the stigma of HIV disease is unlikely to decrease significantly. Nevertheless, it does show some signs of diminishing. Although myths about the casual transmission of HIV remain common, the proportion of people holding such beliefs has diminished with time. Concurrently, as gay men become a smaller proportion of all persons with HIV disease, its image as a "gay disease" is declining. Along with this decline should come a partial reduction in the blame attached to persons with this illness. In addition, as the years pass, HIV disease is losing its aura as an especially mysterious illness. Scientific understanding of HIV disease continues to grow, and news coverage is increasingly making this illness a part of the natural landscape, rather than something inherently different and alien. Consequently, in future, persons who develop HIV disease may receive more humane responses from others than has been the case to date.

Truly significant change in the social construction of HIV disease, however, will not happen until scientists develop a cure or fully effective treatment. The prospects for this are not good.[30] The same lack of knowledge about HIV and problems with developing such knowledge that hinder the search for a vaccine also hinder the search for treatments. In addition, few treatments exist for any viral diseases, and almost none for retroviruses. As a result, scientists lack useful models on which to draw in developing treatments for HIV disease.

Moreover, the nature of HIV makes it an especially difficult virus to control once in the body. Like other retroviruses, but unlike other, more common, sorts of viruses, HIV becomes an integral part of the DNA of every bodily cell it infects. Consequently, most drugs strong enough to kill HIV will also kill the bodies' normal cells, producing intolerable nausea, anemia, or other side effects. In addition, unlike most other viruses, HIV can cross what is called the blood-brain barrier and infect brain cells. Most antiviral drugs, however, cannot cross that barrier. As a result, these drugs cannot halt HIV once it reaches the brain; zidovudine has raised so many hopes and proven relatively effective because it is one of the few exceptions.

Nevertheless, optimism about the potential for treating HIV disease has grown enormously. Entering the 1990s, some, especially HIV activists, clinicians, and government spokespersons, now refer to HIV disease as a chronic and manageable, rather than fatal, illness. They base their optimism on recent research into the effects of zidovudine and newer antiviral drugs such as ddI (dideoxyinosine) and ddC (dideoxycytidine). Early research on zidovudine had suggested that the drug could extend the life span of persons with full-blown AIDS. Preliminary research now suggests that, at least during the relatively brief time period covered by these studies, persons in the early stages of HIV disease are less likely to develop severe HIV disease or AIDS if they take zidovudine. Moreover, zidovudine seems to have fewer side effects when given to persons at earlier stages of HIV disease than when given to persons with AIDS. This research also indicates that rotating zidovudine with other drugs and giving it in lower dosages can decrease its side effects without decreasing its effectiveness. Furthermore, some who cannot tolerate zidovudine can tolerate one of the newer drugs, lending hope that every person with HIV disease will be able to find some drug to extend his or her life span.

Other observers, however, especially bench scientists who are more detached from persons with HIV disease, remain far more pessimistic. These observers argue that, in the words of Jeffrey Levi, an activist and Washington lobbyist for Gay Men's Health Crisis, "People's rhetoric has gotten a little ahead of the science."[31] They believe that although persons with HIV disease will live longer in the future than in the past, they will not live normal life spans and will still die as a result of HIV. In addition, those who take a pessimistic view argue that current research findings do not support the belief that any watershed has been passed in the treatment of HIV. They note, for example, that some persons with HIV disease become resistant to zidovudine and suggest that if individuals begin taking the drug at earlier stages, they will have more time to become resistant. Consequently, zidovudine may help them ward off early, minor health problems but prove ineffective at later stages when they develop more serious opportunistic infections. In addition, those who take a more pessimistic view note that none of the available research can tell us whether these drugs will increase the average life span of persons with HIV disease.[32] The existing studies have only looked at what happens to individuals during brief time periods. During those periods, individuals who take zidovudine are less likely to develop AIDS or to die than those who do not. Over a longer span of time, however, the latter may be just as likely to die. The only difference may be that they either will not develop AIDS before dying or will develop AIDS closer to the time of death.

The difference between these two viewpoints is not as great as it may seem, however. When pressed, many who describe HIV as a chronic illness will also add that it is, of course, still fatal. All agree that the life spans of persons with HIV disease who have sufficient money and information will increase as a result of improvements in treatments. And all agree that millions of persons with HIV disease around the world will continue to die because they lack these resources. In large part, then, the difference between the optimists and the pessimists is that the former believe that in the near future, death from HIV disease will no longer occur shortly after symptoms begin, but, like death from diabetes or some forms of cancer, will occur ten or twenty years after individuals' health begins to deteriorate.

The debate regarding the nature of HIV disease is not simply an intellectual one. Indeed, probably one reason this debate has become so heated is that both sides realize its many significant, practical consequences.

Currently, many people defer obtaining a diagnosis of HIV

disease until they are seriously ill because they fear learning that they have what seems an incurable and fatal illness. If HIV disease is redefined as a chronic and manageable condition, at least some of these individuals will seek diagnosis and treatment earlier. In turn, this will help lengthen their lives.

Such a change in the definition of HIV disease will also change somewhat the responses of others to those who have this illness. Currently, many vocational rehabilitation agencies and other such programs will not work with persons who have HIV disease, on the grounds that it is not worth investing time and energy to help someone who will die soon anyway. If the belief grows that such persons can still expect to live many years (although not necessarily a normal life span), this policy will change and the services available to them will improve.

Redefining HIV disease as a chronic illness will also help protect individuals from other forms of discrimination. Currently, many employers, landlords, and others believe it is safe to discriminate against persons with HIV disease, because, they assume, these persons will die or become incapacitated before they could successfully sue. If it begins to seem that such persons will live long enough to file successful suits, lawyers will become more willing to take on such cases and potential discriminators less willing to risk one.

The redefinition of HIV disease as a chronic, manageable illness also carries potential dangers with it, however. Such a redefinition could encourage the government to restrict funding for research and education on the grounds that HIV disease is no more deserving of special resources or attention than any other illness; some of the more jaundiced observers speculate that this is why government bureaucrats have been especially quick to hail all the recent advances in HIV research. At the same time, insurance companies may become even less willing to pay for the care of persons with HIV disease if they believe that care will continue indefinitely, rather than for only a few years. In addition, those who are at risk for HIV may become less responsive to messages about preventing its spread if infection no longer seems such a devastating prospect. Finally, those who already are infected and who adopt optimistic interpretations of HIV disease may suffer increased emotional strain as their image of the future crumbles and may suffer practical difficulties if they have made plans on the assumptions that their health would not decline. Thus, whether the illness is redefined as chronic and manageable or retains its current definition as fatal, those who live with HIV disease will still face a difficult future.

Conclusions

Making a life with any serious, chronic illness is difficult. However, both the biology of HIV disease and its social construction make it especially devastating. All illnesses evoke some degree of fear in people. Because of its sudden appearance and deadliness, however, and because of still-unanswered questions about its natural history, HIV disease evokes especially great dread in many people—from doctors and nurses to members of the public to those who are themselves ill. Similarly, to some extent the public always considers ill persons to blame for their illnesses. Because HIV disease was first identified among gay men and intravenous drug users, however, the idea that people who have this illness deserve it is especially widespread and entrenched. Consequently, persons with HIV disease must cope simultaneously with a progressive, apparently fatal illness that causes physical and mental disability and with tremendous social stigma. This book has documented the physical and social damage wrought by HIV disease and the varied ways individuals struggle to make a meaningful life for themselves and to maintain their self-concepts as worthwhile human beings despite this illness.

The changes we can expect in the next decade are at least as likely to worsen as to better the situation of persons with HIV disease. Earlier diagnosis, for example, will enable individuals to receive prophylactic treatment earlier, but will also subject them to earlier poverty and stigma. Similarly, the spread of HIV disease should help reduce some of its stigma by reducing the connection in people's minds between the illness and gay men, but it will also result in further overburdening our health care system and lowering the quality of care available to those who fall ill. Even those anticipated changes that appear to promise the most hope have their dark sides; as the life span of persons with HIV disease lengthens, for example, insurance companies may become even more loath to provide care.

In the areas where HIV has hit the hardest, few can still claim to be untouched by this illness. Very soon, we will *all* know someone who has HIV disease—a friend, relative, lover, child. Or we may find that we ourselves are infected. In either event, we will be forced to change how we view and respond to ourselves and our world. Our measure as individuals and as a society will be judged by how we meet this challenge.

Personal Reflections on Researching HIV Disease

During my "apprenticeship" as a sociologist, both during and after graduate school, I was taught how to review the literature, conduct interviews, analyze data, and the like. By the time I began this book, I had been out of graduate school and working as a sociologist for eight years. Nevertheless, in all those years, nothing I had read and no one I had studied with had taught me how to deal with the personal, legal, and ethical dilemmas I encountered while interviewing persons with HIV disease for this book.

Personal Dilemmas

When I began this research, I expected it to be psychologically draining. In retrospect, however, I was terribly naive about the stresses I would encounter.

My most serious problem has been the unusually burdensome sense of responsibility this research created. Probably all researchers struggle with doubts about their abilities to do justice to their topics, particularly when others have provided financial support. However, the nature of my work has heightened this sense of responsibility enormously. If my research becomes widely read, it may affect health care policy and hence significantly affect many individuals' lives. Already, for example, I have testified to our

Governor's Task Force on AIDS, and have learned that my testimony was influential in convincing the task force to oppose mandatory reporting of persons who test positive for HIV. More crucially, in terms of its personal emotional impact, many people I spoke with explicitly referred to their interviews as legacies. They participated in this project despite the emotional and sometimes physical pain it caused them because they believed I would use their stories to help others. Thus they gave me the responsibility of giving meaning to their lives and to their deaths.

I also have encountered personal difficulties in doing this research because it has made the inevitability of death and the possibility of disability far more salient for me. Early in the research, I realized that at each interview I automatically compared my age with that of the person I was interviewing. I was frequently disturbed to find that they were much younger than they looked and often younger than I. (I was thirty-four when I began this research.) Having to witness the pain of their lives was far more difficult than coping with the knowledge that they were dying, especially because the dying occurred out of my sight.

In addition to teaching me some truths about death and disability, the interviews also forced me to recognize the irrational nature of my own and others' response to potential contagion. To control my fears during interviews with those who have HIV disease, I often found myself repeating silently a calming litany about how HIV is and isn't transmitted. Meanwhile, I had to calm the fears of friends and acquaintances who wondered whether I had become a source of contagion. All I could do was to provide information about HIV, which they might or might not choose to assimilate. Fortunately, no one proved irrationally fearful.

Legal Dilemmas

I initially became involved in research on HIV disease after hearing a lecture about how the government is restricting the civil liberties of persons with this illness. These restrictions include deporting noncitizens and quarantining those judged a danger to themselves or others. I was therefore sensitized to the potential legal problems before I began this research. This was an issue from the start because Arizona law requires all health care workers to report to the state any person who has HIV disease at any stage. According to the state department of health services, I could legally be required to report anyone I interviewed (several of whom told me they had not been reported by their doctors). Moreover, an important recent case had confirmed that sociologists' rights to protect their data against subpoenas is not as strong as the right granted to physicians or lawyers.[1] Consequently, and recognizing that reporting someone could jeopardize their civil rights, I was unusually concerned about protecting the confidentiality of my records.

The need for confidentiality produced some unexpected difficulties. I wanted to make it easy for persons with HIV disease who were considering participating in this research to reach me, because I assumed that any difficulty might diminish their willingness to do so. However, I could not give out my home phone number because my housemate might listen to our answering machine and unintentionally hear a message meant only for me. Similarly, I could not write names, addresses, or phone numbers in the pocket calendar that I use to organize my life because I could not risk having the calendar subpoenaed and losing all my other daily records.

Ironically, my chief worry was protecting the signed "informed consent forms" that my university's research ethics committee required me to obtain from each person I interviewed. When I initially raised this issue with the committee, we were unable to reach an agreement on an alternative that would not require individuals to sign their names. (When, in 1989, I began interviewing persons with HIV disease again, however, we agreed that instead of having each sign a consent form, I would begin each interview by reading a statement about informed consent and would tape both my statement and their response.)

Ethical Dilemmas

Early in my training as a sociologist, I learned the value of informed consent. Translating this principle into action, however, requires more than simply presenting potential interviewees with a description of one's purposes and research methods. While interviewing persons with HIV disease, I soon discovered that many assumed that I was a counselor, worked for one of the community organizations that helps persons with HIV disease, or was a lesbian. I then had to decide how much responsibility I had to correct their assumptions, particularly when they were not explicit. Should I have assumed that they understood what a sociologist was, or should I have carefully differentiated sociology from social work? If an individual commented that I did not wear a wedding ring, should I have assumed that they were searching for a polite way of asking if I was a lesbian? How many times should I have stopped a given interview to explain that I did not work for a community organization, if the person I was interviewing did not understand the first time I explained?

Truly informed consent was even more rare among those who felt they could not afford to refuse to participate. Despite my disclaimers, many individuals obviously believed I worked for either the state or a community organization for persons with HIV disease. As a result, they may have feared that they would jeopardize their access to services if they did not participate. Even if they believed they would not be punished for lack of cooperation, they may still have believed they would be rewarded for helping. Several, for example, mentioned that they wanted their physicians to consider them exemplary patients so that the physicians would remember them when choosing patients for experimental treatment programs.

Truly free consent was even less likely in interviewing individuals who were in jail or prison. Because of the connection between HIV and drug use, many persons with HIV disease are imprisoned. As a result, I initially pursued the possibility of contacting persons with HIV disease through the health department of the state prison system. My first contacts with prison officials seemed promising. Even more than other persons with HIV disease, however, prisoners might have felt that they would be punished if they refused to participate. Moreover, I would have had no way to keep the administration from knowing who had refused, because I would have had to arrange the interviews through prison officials. Consequently, I was relieved when negotiations fell through.

Finally, I faced a broad range of ethical dilemmas when either the persons I interviewed or I myself viewed me as an information or counseling source. Often persons I interviewed asked me questions about the disease, drugs, or doctors. Similarly, I frequently encountered persons with HIV disease whose knowledge of their illness was clearly deficient. I then had to decide whether to answer their questions even if doing so might jeopardize my relationship with influential physicians (who, for example, had not provided information about the side effects of certain drugs). Similarly, I had to decide whether to correct individuals' information if not asked. These questions posed minimal problems compared to those generated by implicit or explicit pleas for counseling. I had no answer for the individual who asked me how to convince her uninfected husband to use condoms. Nor was it clear to me how to respond when individuals told me that their disease was punishment for their sins, or that they felt suicidal, or that their greatest grief was losing their children but they would not contact them for fear of infecting them. Saying nothing did not feel ethical to me. Yet saying something required me to break professional norms for sociological research.

Searching for Solutions

The legal dilemmas posed by this research presented the fewest difficulties, because the problems and solutions were purely practical. To avoid writing confidential information in my usual daily calendar, I began carrying a small notepad with me. As is typical in this sort of research, all my records and tapes were number-coded, and all identifying information was removed from the transcripts and resulting publications (including this book). I recorded data on individuals' age, marital status, occupation, and the like separately from the taped interviews, so that persons who transcribed the tapes would not have that information. I hoped that this would make it more difficult for the transcriptionist to recognize the person I was interviewing, should the transcriptionist happen to know him or her. All papers with names or addresses were kept in one less-than-obvious location and have now been destroyed. In addition, I decided that if I were subpoenaed, I would refuse to turn over the information. (Of course, such a decision is easy to make in the abstract and I cannot predict what I might have done if actually faced with a jail sentence for contempt of court.) Finally, when some individuals, far from desiring confidentiality, told me that they would like me to use their real names in this "legacy" we were creating, I decided not to do so because the potential "stigma fallout" seemed an unfair burden to thrust on unsuspecting friends and relatives.

The remaining problems had no easy answers. I tried to answer all questions, whether direct or indirect, asked by those I interviewed. I also tried to clarify their understanding of such things as sociology versus social work and working *with* versus working *for* a community organization. If someone still seemed not to understand after two or three attempts at explaining, I did not pursue the matter.

When it came to a choice between being ethical and being "sociological," I went with ethical every time. I felt a strong moral obligation to answer any question I was asked and to provide needed information even when not asked directly. I did try to wait until after the individual had finished stating his views before interjecting any information. And I occasionally requested that individuals not tell their doctors that I was their source.

Similarly, I believe it is wrong to listen to a person's feelings of guilt and self-deprecation without attempting to alleviate those feelings. Thus if a person told me he felt horribly stupid for not using "safe sex" until a couple of years ago, I heard him out and then gently suggested that until recently no one knew how HIV was transmitted. I also volunteered suggestions about sources of information and social support when it seemed warranted. I realize that these tactics may have diminished my credibility as a researcher, but I thought that was less important than diminishing my credibility as a person.

Finally, I did whatever I could to maintain my own mental health, because I realized I would be of little use to anyone if I allowed myself to burn out. So I tried to restrict my contacts with those who have HIV disease to interviews. This tactic proved insufficient on two notable occasions—once when the family of someone I interviewed, recognizing that the interview had been an important experience for their relative, asked me if I would visit him on his deathbed, and the second time when students asked me to speak at a memorial vigil for an alumnus who had recently died of HIV disease. Finishing this book, especially given my fairly pessimistic predictions for the future, has been made much more difficult because I now have one good friend with HIV disease.

For my sanity's sake, I was grateful that at the time I was conducting most of these interviews I had no friends in high-risk groups (so far as I knew), that I did not know what any of the people I interviewed were like before their illness, and that I did not have to see them as their health deteriorated. For this reason I was very reluctant to do follow-up interviews, even though I knew they would provide invaluable data; it took many months of soul-searching before I felt able to do so. Similarly, for a long time I avoided taking any steps that would have committed me to continuing this research for more than a year at a time. Knowing that my commitment was finite made it far more manageable psychologically.

I also learned the hard way that it was much more difficult emotionally for me to interview women than to interview men, because I identified so much more strongly wtih the women. The summer I began interviewing women was the summer I began having nightmares about contracting HIV disease. Fortunately for my mental health, although not for my research project, few women with HIV disease were available for interviews in Arizona.

To protect my mental and physical health, I tried always to schedule my interviews so that I would have time for exercise afterward, and tried to satisfy my worries with popcorn rather than chocolate. I calmed other new anxieties by updating my will, obtaining disability insurance, and giving a friend a medical power of attorney. I also soon lost most of my inhibitions about discussing the research and my attendant emotions, for I learned that it helped to share the burden. I remember vividly one afternoon when I stopped a casual acquaintance in a supermarket and harangued him for about forty minutes with my troubles. He felt worse afterward, but I felt much better.

Undoubtedly many other researchers have coped with similar problems over the years. Unfortunately, norms for professional conduct do not allow easy and open discussion with colleagues about either psychological or ethical problems, while the rarity of lawsuits leaves few of us sensitized to legal issues. As a result, many universities provide excellent technical training in research skills, but few prepare students for dealing with these nontechnical but equally crucial difficulties. I am sure that I reinvented the wheel in my attempts to deal with these dilemmas, but I found few good places to read about—let alone discuss—my concerns. In the long run, the unusual stresses of research on HIV disease may have at least one serendipitous effect, if they pressure scholars to begin tackling these issues openly.

APPENDIX 2

Methodology

This appendix describes the persons I interviewed for this book, how I contacted them, and the methods I used to analyze the data.

Sampling PWAs and Their Doctors

The data for this book come from three sets of interviews: two with persons who have HIV disease and one with their doctors. In 1986 and 1987, I interviewed twenty-five Arizona residents who had been diagnosed with AIDS or ARC. I reinterviewed thirteen of these individuals four to six months later. (Two respondents declined to participate in the follow-up interviews, two moved without leaving an address, and eight died or suffered brain damage in the interim.) Twenty of the twenty-five were men who described themselves as gay or bisexual and who had not used intravenous drugs. The remaining five (two heterosexual women and three gay men) had injected drugs.

At the time of these first interviews, few women in Arizona had been diagnosed with HIV disease. These numbers increased steadily during the time I was working on this book. Because I wanted to see how life with HIV disease might differ for those who are not gay men, and because of my interest in gender issues, I decided in 1989 to do a second set of interviews specifically with women. I subsequently interviewed an additional six women who had AIDS and six who were at earlier stages of HIV disease. Five of the women had become infected through sharing needles and one through a blood transfusion. The rest had become infected through heterosexual intercourse—two with hemophiliacs, three with drug users, and one with a husband who had received a contaminated blood transfusion.

To obtain my samples of persons with HIV disease, I asked the four nonprofit groups in the state that offer emotional and financial support to such persons to mail letters to their clients describing the study. To increase sample size and diversity, I also posted signs in gay bars, published announcements in gay newspapers and the mainstream press, announced the study in political action groups that deal with HIV disease, and asked physicians, drug counselors, HIV disease educators, street outreach workers, and individuals who run support groups for persons with HIV disease to inform their clients of the study. Finally, I asked the people I interviewed to give my name to any other persons with HIV disease whom they knew. No names were given to me by any source. Instead, individuals were invited to contact me if they wanted to participate in the study.

Most of the people I interviewed (twenty-eight of the thirty-seven) learned of this study through letters from the four nonprofit groups. Another two learned of the study from friends, two from a political action group, one from a notice in a gay newspaper, and four through their doctors. Some had experienced almost no health problems, while others had already experienced life-threatening infections. Because participating in an interview required some stamina, however, all persons I spoke with were still relatively healthy. Their ages range from twenty-two to fifty-seven; 62 percent were in their thirties and 27 percent in their twenties. Only 3 percent were Hispanic or black, compared to 13 percent of Arizona AIDS cases.[1]

In addition to interviewing persons with HIV disease, I also interviewed Arizona doctors who treat such persons. To identify such doctors, in 1988 I sent letters describing my proposed research to all infectious disease physicians listed in the state medical directory; all physicians working for the Indian Health Service; all dentists working for government-run clinics; and all physicians and dentists whom political activists, state health department employees, or other respondents believed treated persons with HIV disease. I did not interview any medical residents because they cannot choose who they treat. Nor did I interview doctors who had treated fewer than three persons with HIV disease, because of the odds that those few individuals were the doctors' patients before they became infected rather than new patients the doctors had accepted despite their diagnosis.

Through these methods I identified thirty-seven doctors who had treated three or more persons with HIV disease. Twenty-six of these (70 percent) agreed to be interviewed. Nine of the twenty-six were primary practitioners (in family practice, general practice, or internal medicine), eleven were infectious disease specialists, three were oncologists, and three were dentists. Slightly more than half (54 percent) work alone, while the rest work for hospitals or clinics. Almost one-quarter (23 percent) were working on funded HIV research at the time of the interviews. The total number of persons with HIV disease that each doctor had treated ranged from three to several hundred, the latter figure among those affiliated with university research projects. Just under half (46 percent) had treated three to twenty-five persons with HIV disease; the rest had treated twenty-six or more.

All but two of the doctors are men, and, reflecting the state's demographic patterns, all but one live in the Phoenix or Tucson area. Ages range from thirty-two to sixty-three, with one-third (32 percent) under age forty. Sixteen describe themselves as heterosexual, six as homosexual, and one as bisexual; three declined to answer the question. Seven doctors (including one heterosexual doctor) believe that they are "known in the gay community as good doctors for gay people to go to."

Data Collection and Analysis

All the interviews, with doctors and with those who have HIV disease, were semi-structured. I entered each interview with a preset list of questions, but also probed into any areas that emerged as potentially significant during the course of the interview. Initial interviews with persons who have HIV disease ranged from two to five hours in length and averaged about three hours; follow-up interviews were considerably shorter. Interviews with doctors averaged about one hour. All interviews but one were audiotaped and transcribed. (One doctor preferred that I hand-record my notes.) Interviews with persons who have HIV disease took place at their homes and those with doctors at their doctors' offices unless they preferred another location (usually my home). I attempted to ask all questions and respond to all answers in an unbiased and non-judgmental manner, whether my respondent was describing sado-masochistic homosexual behaviors or fundamentalist Christian theology. I believe I was successful in that no one I interviewed responded hostilely, broke off the interviews (except from physical exhaustion), or in any other way suggested that they felt uncomfortable discussing these issues with me.

Because my purpose was to understand how the people I interviewed saw their lives, I analyzed the data using categories that emerged from their descriptions of their situations. After each interview, I revised the interview schedule to focus it more closely on these emerging themes. I used subsequent interviews to hone my understanding of these themes. When collapsed and reorganized, these themes formed the structure of the chapters.

Notes

Chapter 1. Introduction

1. To protect the privacy of the people I interviewed, I have changed all names, as well as some identifying information such as occupation.

2. For example, see Kathryn A. Atchison, Theresa A. Dolan, and Harriette K. Meetz, "Have Dentists Assimilated Information About AIDS?," *Journal of Dental Education* 51 (1987):668–672; R. Nathan Link, Anat R. Feingold, Mitchell H. Charap, Katherine Freeman, and Steven P. Shelov, "Concerns of Medical and Pediatric House Officers About Acquiring AIDS from Their Patients," *American Journal of Public Health* 78 (1988):455–459; and Jean L. Richardson, Thomas Lochner, Kimberly McGuignan, and Alexandra M. Levine, "Physician Attitudes and Experience Regarding the Care of Patients with Acquired Immunodeficiency Syndrome (AIDS) and Related Disorders (ARC)," *Medical Care* 25 (1987):675–685.

3. For instance, see Erving Goffman, *Stigma: Notes on the Management of Spoiled Identity* (Englewood Cliffs, N.J.: Prentice-Hall, 1963); and Julius A. Roth, *Timetables* (Indianapolis: Bobbs-Merrill, 1963).

4. See Peter Conrad, "The Experience of Illness: Recent and New Directions," *Research in the Sociology of Health Care* 6 (1987):1–31; and Joseph Schneider and Peter Conrad, *Having Epilepsy: The Experience and Control of Illness* (Philadelphia: Temple University Press, 1983).

5. Reviewed in Conrad, "The Experience of Illness."

6. Centers for Disease Control, *HIV/AIDS Surveillance Report* (December 1989).

7. Figures obtained from Arizona Department of Health Services, *Definitive and Presumptive AIDS cases in Arizona and AIDS Related Complex (ARC): Surveillance Report for Arizona* (December 1988), and from Centers

for Disease Control, "AIDS and Human Immunodeficiency Virus Infection in the United States: 1988 Update," *Morbidity and Mortality Weekly Report* 38, no. S-4(1989).

Chapter 2. Social Construction of HIV Disease

1. "Pneumocystis Pneumonia—Los Angeles," *Morbidity and Mortality Weekly Report* 30, no. 21 (1981):250–252.

2. "Kaposi's Sarcoma and Pneumocystis Pneumonia Among Homosexual Men—New York and California," *Morbidity and Mortality Weekly Report* 30, no. 25 (1981):305–308.

3. Described in Ronald Bayer, *Private Acts, Social Consequences: AIDS and the Politics of Public Health* (New York: Free Press, 1989), pp. 72–80; and Randy Shilts, *And the Band Played On: Politics, People, and the AIDS Epidemic* (New York: St. Martin's Press, 1987).

4. Figures obtained from U.S. General Accounting Office, *AIDS Forecasting: Undercount of Cases and Lack of Key Data Weaken Existing Estimates* GAO/PEMD-89-13 (Washington, D.C.: Government Printing Office, 1989); and World Health Organization, *Update: AIDS Cases Reported to Surveillance, Forecasting and Impact Assessment Unit (SFI)* (1 June 1989).

5. See Stephen O. Murray and Kenneth W. Payne, "Medical Policy Without Scientific Evidence: The Promiscuity Paradigm and AIDS," *California Sociologist* 11 (1988):13–54.

6. U.S. General Accounting Office, *AIDS Forecasting,* p. 56.

7. Murray and Payne, "Medical Policy Without Scientific Evidence."

8. Gerald M. Oppenheimer, "In the Eye of the Storm: The Epidemiological Construction of AIDS," in Elizabeth Fee and Daniel M. Fox, eds., *AIDS: The Burdens of History,* (Berkeley and Los Angeles: University of California Press, 1988), pp. 267–300.

9. Mary O'Donnell, "Lesbian Health Care: Issues and Literature," *Science for the People* (May/June 1978):8–15.

10. William L. Heyward and James W. Curran, "The Epidemiology of AIDS in the U.S.," *Scientific American* 259, no. 4 (1988):72–81.

11. Figures obtained from Centers for Disease Control, *HIV/AIDS Surveillance Report.* No mode of transmission has been identified for 3 per-

cent of AIDS cases. These cases involve people who died before they were interviewed, refused to answer questions posed by government researchers, or did not know conclusively if any of their heterosexual partners had been infected with HIV.

12. Jean Seligmann with Ruth Marshall, "Checking up on a Killer: A Grim Report on the AIDS Toll for the 1990s," *Newsweek,* 12 June 1989, p. 59.

13. Heyward and Curran, "The Epidemiology of AIDS in the U.S.," p. 80.

14. See, for example, the Walter Reed staging system described in Robert R. Redfield and Donald S. Burke, "HIV Infection: The Clinical Picture," *Scientific American* 259, no. 4 (1988):90–98.

15. For discussions of the media's treatment of HIV disease, see Andrea J. Baker, "The Portrayal of AIDS in the Media: An Analysis of Articles in the *New York Times,*" in Douglas A. Feldman and Thomas M. Johnson, eds., *The Social Dimensions of AIDS: Methods and Theory* (New York: Praeger, 1986), pp. 179–197; William A. Check, "Beyond the Political Model of Reporting: Nonspecific Symptoms in Media Communication About AIDS," *Reviews of Infectious Diseases* 9 (1987):987–1000; Larry Kramer, *Reports from the Holocaust: The Making of an AIDS Activist* (New York: St. Martin's Press, 1989); James Kinsella, "How to Cover a Plague," in Richard A. Berk, ed., *The Social Impact of AIDS in the U.S.* (Cambridge, Mass.: Abt Books, 1988), pp. 115–122; Sandra Panem, *The AIDS Bureaucracy* (Cambridge, Mass.: Harvard University Press, 1988); and Shilts, *And the Band Played On.*

16. My thanks to Diane Wysocki for these statistics.

17. This process is described in Shilts, *And the Band Played On,* and in Baker, "The Portrayal of AIDS." For an example, see Michael Ver Meulen, "The Gay Plague," *New York* 15 (31 May 1982):52–61.

18. Edward Albert, "Illness and Deviance: The Response of the Press to AIDS," in Feldman and Johnson, eds., *The Social Dimensions of AIDS,* pp. 163–178.

19. "The Acquired Immune Deficiency Syndrome," *Journal of the American Medical Association* 249 (1983):2375.

20. Shilts, *And the Band Played On.*

21. Albert, "Illness and Deviance," pp. 174–175.

22. William Check, a medical journalist and former microbiologist, provides an excellent analysis of how the basic nature of journalism

contributed to the media's poor coverage of HIV disease in "Beyond the Political Model of Reporting."

23. Check, "Beyond the Political Model of Reporting."

24. William Masters, Virginia Johnson, and Robert Kolodny, *Crisis: Heterosexual Behavior in the Age of AIDS* (New York: Grove Press, 1988), p. 7.

25. Ibid., p. 94.

26. National Center for Health Statistics, A. M. Hardy and D. A. Dawson, "AIDS Knowledge and Attitudes for October and November 1988: Provisional Data from the National Health Interview Survey," *Advance Data from Vital and Health Statistics* No. 167. DHHS Pub. No (PHS) 89-1250 (Hyattsville, Md.: Public Health Service, 1989).

27. Charles F. Turner, Heather G. Miller, and Lincoln E. Moses, eds., *AIDS: Sexual Behavior and Intravenous Drug Use* (Washington, D.C.: National Academy Press, 1989), p. 394.

28. George Gallup, *The Gallup Poll: Public Opinion 1982* (Wilmington, Del.: Scholarly Resources, 1983), pp. 253, 266–269.

29. Joseph R. Gusfield, *Symbolic Crusade: Status Politics and the American Temperance Movement* (Urbana, Il.: University of Illinois Press, 1963).

30. "AIDS is a Moral Issue," in *AIDS: Opposing Viewpoints,* Lynn Hall and Thomas Modl, eds. (St. Paul, Minn.: Greenhaven Press, 1988), pp. 34–35.

31. "AIDS, Nature and the Nature of AIDS," *National Review* 37, no. 21 (1 November 1985):18.

32. Gene Antonio, *The AIDS Cover-Up? The Real and Alarming Facts About AIDS* (San Francisco: Ignatius Press, 1986).

33. "Fundamentalists Call AIDS God's Plague on Gays," *Arizona Republic,* 25 November 1989, p. G2.

34. See, for example, Antonio, *The AIDS Cover-Up,* pp. 77–81; and Enrique T. Rueda and Michael Schwartz, *Gays, AIDS and You* (Old Greenwich, Conn.: Devin Adair, 1987).

35. Rueda and Schwartz, *Gays, AIDS, and You,* pp. 7–8.

36. 131 *Congressional Record* H7986, 1 October 1985.

37. Antonio, *The AIDS Cover-Up,* p. xii.

38. Antonio, *The AIDS Cover-Up,* p. 147.

39. See, for example, Antonio, *The AIDS Cover-Up;* and Joseph Sobran, "The Politics of AIDS," *National Review* 38, no. 9 (23 May 1986):22–26 + .

40. Centers for Disease Control, *HIV/AIDS Surveillance Report*.

41. This discussion draws heavily on Steve Connor and Sharon Kingman, *The Search for the Virus: The Scientific Discovery of AIDS and the Quest for a Cure* (London: Penguin Books, 1988); Renee Sabatier, *Blaming Others: Prejudice, Race, and Worldwide AIDS* (London: Panos Institute, 1988); and Renee Sabatier, *AIDS and the Third World* (London: Panos Institute, 1989).

42. Gallup, *The Gallup Poll: Public Opinion 1987* (Wilmington, Del.: Scholarly Resources, 1988), pp. 260–271.

43. Los Angeles *Times* Poll, Study #126, 1987.

44. Rodney G. Triplet and David B. Sugarman, "Reactions to AIDS Victims: Ambiguity Breeds Contempt," *Personality and Social Psychology Bulletin* 13 (1987):265–274.

45. Irwin Katz, R. Glen Hass, Nina Parisi, Janetta Astone, and Denise McEvaddy, "Lay People's and Health Care Personnel's Perceptions of Cancer, AIDS, Cardiac, and Diabetic Patients," *Psychological Reports* 60 (1987):615–629.

46. Triplet and Sugarman, "Reactions to AIDS Victims."

47. David Lester, "Prejudice Toward AIDS Patients Versus Other Terminally Ill Patients," *American Journal of Public Health* 78 (1988):854.

48. Robert Steinbrook, "AIDS Fear Drops, Attitudes Harden," Los Angeles *Times,* 16 July 1989, p. A1+.

49. Los Angeles *Times* Poll, Study #126, 1987.

50. For an excellent discussion of the interplay between politics and public health responses to HIV disease, see Bayer, *Private Acts, Social Consequences*.

51. Ibid., pp. 137–158.

52. These studies are reviewed in Horst Stipp and Dennis Kerr, "Determinants of Public Opinion About AIDS," *Public Opinion Quarterly* 53 (1989):98–106. To the best of my knowledge, no study has correlated attitudes toward HIV disease with attitudes toward either drug use or nonwhites.

53. Stephen D. Johnson, "Factors Related to Intolerance of AIDS Victims," *Journal for the Scientific Study of Religion* 26 (1987):105–110.

54. Shilts, *And the Band Played On*, provides a vivid, if nonscholarly, account of the government's response—or lack of response—to the emergence of HIV.

55. Panem, *The AIDS Bureaucracy*, p. 29; and Bayer, *Private Acts, Social Consequences*, pp. 158–165.

56. Shilts, *And the Band Played On.*

57. U.S. Congress, Office of Technology Assessment, *Review of the Public Health Service's Response to AIDS: A Technical Memorandum* OTA-TM-H-24, (Washington, D.C.: OTA, 1985).

58. Panem, *The AIDS Bureaucracy,* p. 95.

59. #88-436-P (Washington, D.C.: Government Printing Office, (24 June 1988).

60. Shilts, *And the Band Played On,* p. 186.

61. U.S. Congress, *Review of the Public Health Service's Response to AIDS.*

62. P.L. 100-436 at 102 Stat. 1692.

63. Centers for Disease Control, *Program Announcement and Notice of Availability of Funds for Fiscal Year 1986,* p. 18. Emphasis mine.

64. *Congressional Record,* 14 October 1987, S-14217.

65. Jane H. Aiken, "Education as Prevention," in Harlon L. Dalton, Scott Burris, and the Yale AIDS Law Project, eds., *AIDS and the Law: A Guide for the Public* (New Haven: Yale University Press, 1987), pp. 90–105.

66. The courts' response to HIV disease is reviewed in Arthur S. Leonard, "AIDS in the Workplace," in Dalton, Burris, and the Yale AIDS Law Project, eds., *AIDS and the Law: A Guide for the Public,* pp. 109–125.

Chapter 3. The Moral Status of Illness

1. Peter Conrad and Joseph W. Schneider, *Deviance and Medicalization: From Badness to Sickness* (St. Louis: Mosby, 1980), p. 36.

2. American Society of Plastic and Reconstructive Surgeons, *Comments on the Proposed Classification of Inflatable Breast Prosthesis and Silicone Gel Filled Breast Prosthesis* (1 July 1989), pp. 4–5.

3. For example, see J. M. Burger, "Motivational Biases in the Attribution of Responsibility for an Accident: A Meta-Analysis of the Defensive-Attribution Hypothesis," *Psychological Bulletin* 90 (1981):496–512; M. J. Lerner and D. T. Miller, "Just World Research and the Attribution Process: Looking Back and Ahead," *Psychological Bulletin* 85 (1978):1030–1051; and Beth E. Meyerowitz, Janice G. Williams, and Jocelyne Gessner, "Perceptions of Controllability and Attitudes Toward

Cancer and Cancer Patients," *Journal of Applied Social Psychology* 17 (1987):471–492.

4. George Foster, "Disease Etiologies in Non-western Medical Systems," *American Anthropologist* 78 (1976):773–782.

5. George P. Murdock, *Theories of Illness: A World Survey* (Pittsburgh: University of Pittsburgh Press, 1980).

6. Ibid., pp. 42–52.

7. Robert S. Gottfried, *The Black Death: Natural and Human Disaster in Medieval Europe* (New York: Free Press, 1983), provides an excellent history of the plague.

8. Ibid., pp. 110–115; and Michael W. Dols, *The Black Death in the Middle East* (Princeton, N.J.: Princeton University Press, 1977), p. 89.

9. Dols, *The Black Death,* p. 23.

10. Ibid., p. 113.

11. Researchers now believe that the "leprosy" described in the Bible is not the same as what we currently call leprosy. Rather, the Hebrew term *tsaraat* and the Greek term *lepra* (used in the Old and New Testaments, respectively) referred to a wide variety of skin disorders; leprosy may not even have been among them since archeological evidence suggests that it did not exist until about 300 B.C.E. This evidence is discussed in Stanley G. Browne, "Leprosy in the Bible," in Bernard Palmer, ed., *Medicine and the Bible* (Exeter, U.K.: Paternoster Press, 1986), pp. 101–125. Nevertheless, for many centuries these biblical writings provided the context for social responses to persons with what was considered leprosy. In an attempt to reduce the stigma of leprosy by breaking the connection between the biblical and modern illnesses, some public health workers and activists now refer to leprosy as Hansen's disease, after the doctor who first identified the causative microorganism.

12. Peter Richards, *The Medieval Leper and his Northern Heirs* (Totowa, N.J.: Rowman & Littlefield, 1977), pp. 123–124.

13. Zachary Gussow and George S. Tracy, "Stigma and the Leprosy Phenomenon: The Social History of a Disease in the Nineteenth and Twentieth Centuries," *Bulletin of the History of Medicine* 44 (1970):425–449.

14. Stanley Stein, *Alone No Longer* (New York: Funk and Wagnalls, 1963).

15. See ibid., and Perry Burgess, *Who Walk Alone* (New York: Holt, 1940).

16. Charles E. Rosenberg, "Disease and Social Order in America: Perceptions and Expectations," in Elizabeth Fee and Daniel M. Fox, eds., *AIDS: The Burdens of History* (Berkeley: and Los Angeles University of California Press, 1988), pp. 12–32.

17. Rosenberg, *The Cholera Years: The United States in 1832, 1849, and 1866* (Chicago: University of Chicago Press, 1962, rev. 1987); and Guenter B. Risse, "Epidemics and History: Ecological Perspectives and Social Responses," in Fee and Fox, eds. *AIDS: The Burdens of History,* pp. 33–66.

18. Risse, "Epidemics and History," p. 45.

19. Described in Risse, "Epidemics and History"; Rosenberg, *The Cholera Years;* and Rosenberg, "Disease and Social Order."

20. For example, see Mildred Blaxter, "The Causes of Disease: Women Talking," *Social Science and Medicine* 17 (1983):59–69; Cecil G. Helman, " 'Feed a Cold, Starve a Fever,': Folk Models of Infection in an English Suburban Community, and Their Relation to Medical Treatment," in Caroline Currer and Meg Stacey, eds., *Concepts of Health, Illness and Disease: A Comparative Perspective* (Leamington Spa, U.K.: Berg, 1986), pp. 211–232; R. Pill and N. Scott, "Concepts of Illness Causation and Responsibility: Some Preliminary Data from a Sample of Working Class Mothers," *Social Science and Medicine* 16 (1982):43–52; and Irving K. Zola, "Medicine as an Institution of Social Control," *Sociological Review* 20 (1972):487–504.

21. Helman, " 'Feed a Cold,' " p. 219.

22. Sylvia Tesh, *Hidden Arguments: Political Ideology and Disease Prevention Policy* (New Brunswick, N.J.: Rutgers University Press, 1988).

23. Michelle Lodge, "How to Heal Yourself," *Ladies' Home Journal* 56 (June 1989):108–111; and Dianne Hales, "Superimmunity: How to Get It," *Woman's Day* (31 May 1988):54–61.

24. For an important analysis of this topic, especially as it relates to cancer and tuberculosis, see Susan Sontag, *Illness as Metaphor* (New York: Farrar, Straus, and Giroux, 1978).

25. Joseph P. Kahn, "Radner's Humor Good Medicine, Even Though It Couldn't Save Her," *Arizona Daily Star,* 30 May 1989, pp. 1C–2C.

26. For a review of these studies, see Aron W. Siegman and Theodore M. Dembroski, eds., *In Search of Coronary Prone Behavior: Beyond Type A* (Hillsdale, N.J.: Lawrence Erlbaum Associates, 1989).

27. Bernie Siegel, *Love, Medicine and Miracles* (New York: Harper and Row, 1986). Marketing figures given in Lodge, "How to Heal Yourself," 1989.

28. For further discussion, see Robert Crawford, "Individual Responsibility and Health Politics," in Susan Reverby and David Rosner, eds., *Health Care in America: Essays in Social History* (Philadelphia: Temple University Press, 1979), pp. 247–268; Howard Waitzkin, "The Social Origins of Illness: A Neglected History," *International Journal of Health Services* 11 (1981):77–103; Tesh, *Hidden Arguments;* and Zola, "Medicine as an Institution of Social Control."

29. Barbara Katz Rothman, *Recreating Motherhood: Ideology and Technology in a Patriarchal Society* (New York: Norton, 1989), p. 21.

30. Peter Conrad, "The Social Meaning of AIDS," *Social Policy* (Summer 1986):51–56.

31. For further discussion, see Allan M. Brandt, *No Magic Bullet: A Social History of Venereal Disease in the United States Since 1880* (New York: Oxford University Press, 1985); Conrad, "The Social Meaning of AIDS"; Karolynn Siegel, "AIDS: The Social Dimension," *Psychiatric Annals* 16 (1986):168–172; and Sontag, *AIDS and Its Metaphors* (New York: Farrar, Straus, and Giroux, 1988), pp. 26–27.

32. David F. Musto, "Quarantine and the Problem of AIDS," in Fee and Fox, eds., *AIDS: The Burdens of History,* pp. 67–85; and James T. Patterson, *The Dread Disease: Cancer and Modern American Culture* (Cambridge, Mass.: Harvard University Press, 1987).

33. Brandt, *No Magic Bullet;* and Jay Cassel, *The Secret Plague: Venereal Disease in Canada, 1838–1939* (Toronto: University of Toronto Press, 1987), pp. 96–97.

34. See Conrad, "The Social Meaning of AIDS."

35. Gussow and Tracy, "Stigma and the Leprosy Phenomenon," p. 427.

36. See Sontag, *AIDS and Its Metaphors,* pp. 38–45.

37. Sontag, *Illness as Metaphor.*

38. See Peter Manning, "Dreadful Disease: A Theory of Illness" (Paper presented at the Michigan Sociological Society, 1983, rev. 1987); and Conrad, "The Social Significance of AIDS."

39. Alfred W. Crosby, Jr., *Epidemic and Peace, 1918* (Westport, Conn.: Greenwood Press, 1976), pp. 207, 311–323.

40. See Sontag, *Illness as Metaphor;* and Manning, "Dreadful Disease."

41. Caroline Myss, *AIDS: Passageway to Transformation* (Walpole, N.H.: Stillpoint Publishing, 1987); Jason Serinus, ed., *Psychoimmunity and the Healing Process: A Holistic Approach to Immunity and AIDS* (Berkeley, Calif.: Celestial Arts, 1986).

42. Louise Hay, *The AIDS Book: Creating a Positive Approach* (Santa Monica, Calif.: Hay House, 1988).

43. Ibid., p. 12.

44. Ibid., p. 13.

45. Ibid., p. 18.

46. My thanks to Barry Adam for helping me conceptualize how the impact of Hay's philosophy might change with the development of the disease. My conclusions, however, are my own, and do not necessarily reflect Adam's views.

Chapter 4. Becoming a Person with HIV Disease

1. See Carol-Ann Emmons et al., "Psychosocial Predictors of Reported Behavior Change in Homosexual Men at Risk for AIDS," *Health Education Quarterly* 13 (1986):331–345; Leon McKusick, William Horstman, and Thomas J. Coates, "AIDS and Sexual Behavior Reported by Gay Men in San Francisco," *American Journal of Public Health* 75(1985):493–496; and Karolynn Siegel, "Patterns of Change in Sexual Behavior Among Gay Men in New York City," *Archives of Sexual Behavior* 17 (1988):481–497.

2. Samuel R. Friedman, Don C. Des Jarlais, and Jo L. Sotheran, "AIDS Health Education for Intravenous Drug Users," *Health Education Quarterly* 13 (1986):383–393; and Harold M. Ginzburg, John French, Joyce Jackson, Peter I. Hartsock, Mhairi Graham MacDonald, and Stanley H. Weiss, "Health Education and Knowledge Assessment of HTLV-III Diseases Among Intravenous Drug Users," *Health Education Quarterly* 13 (1986):373–382.

3. Eleanor Singer, Theresa F. Rogers, and Mary Corcoran, "The Polls—A Report. AIDS," *Public Opinion Quarterly* 51 (1987):580–595.

4. For reviews of the role uncertainty plays in the lives of ill persons, see Peter Conrad, "The Experience of Illness: Recent and New Directions," *Research in the Sociology of Health Care* 6 (1987):1–31; and Barney

G. Glaser and Anselm L. Strauss, *Time for Dying* (Chicago: Aldine, 1968). For discussions of the impact of uncertainty on stress, see Merle H. Mishel, "Perceived Uncertainty and Stress in Illness," *Research in Nursing and Health* 7 (1984):163–171; Merle H. Mishel, Thelma Hostetter, Barbara King, and Vivian Graham, "Predictors of Psychosocial Adjustment in Patients Newly Diagnosed with Gynecological Cancer," *Cancer Nursing* 7 (1984):291–299; and Eric Molleman, Pieter J. Krabbendam, Albertus A. Annyas, Heimen S. Koops, Dirk T. Sleijfer, and Albert Vermey, "The Significance of the Doctor-Patient Relationship in Coping with Cancer," *Social Science and Medicine* 18 (1984):475–480.

5. Diane Beeson, Jane S. Zones and John Nye, "The Social Consequences of AIDS Antibody Testing: Coping with Stigma," (Paper presented at the 1986 Annual Meeting of the Society for the Study of Social Problems, New York); Thomas J. Coates, Stephen Morin, and Leon McKusick, "Behavioral Consequences of AIDS Antibody Testing among Gay Men," *Journal of the American Medical Association* 258 (1987):1889; and J. M. Moulton, "Adjustment to a Diagnosis of AIDS or ARC in Gay Men" (Ph.D. dissertation, California School of Professional Psychology, 1985).

6. Discussed in more detail in Randy Shilts, *And the Band Played On: Politics, People, and the AIDS Epidemic* (New York: St. Martin's Press, 1987); and Ronald Bayer, *Private Acts, Social Consequences: AIDS and the Politics of Public Health* (New York: Free Press, 1989).

7. Karolynn Siegel, Martin P. Levine, Charles Brooks, and Rochelle Kern, "The Motives of Gay Men for Taking or Not Taking the HIV Antibody Test," *Social Problems* 36 (1989):368–383.

8. Compare to ibid.

9. "Human Immune Deficiency Virus Infections," *ACOG Technical Bulletin*, no. 123 (December 1988):1–7.

10. See, for example, Michael Bury, "Chronic Illness as Biographical Disruption," *Sociology of Health and Illness* 4 (1982):167–182; Bill Cowie, "Cardiac Patient's Perception of His Heart Attack," *Social Science and Medicine* 10 (1976):87–96; Joseph W. Schneider and Peter Conrad, *Having Epilepsy: The Experience and Control of Illness* (Philadelphia: Temple University Press, 1983); and David C. Stewart and Thomas J. Sullivan, "Illness Behavior and the Sick Role in Chronic Disease: The Case of Multiple Sclerosis," *Social Science and Medicine* 16 (1982):1397–1404.

11. Charles E. Lewis, Howard E. Freeman, and Christopher R.

Corey, "AIDS-related Competence of California's Primary Care Physicians," *American Journal of Public Health* 77 (1987):795–800.

12. For similar findings with regard to other illnesses, see Bury, "Chronic Illness as Biographical Disruption," p. 172; Stewart and Sullivan, "Illness Behavior and the Sick Role"; Schneider and Conrad, *Having Epilepsy;* and Charles Waddell, "The Process of Neutralisation and the Uncertainties of Cystic Fibrosis," *Sociology of Health and Illness* 4 (1982):210–220.

13. Erving Goffman, *Asylums* (New York: Doubleday, 1961).

14. Peter M. Marzuk, Helen Tierney, and Kenneth Tardiff, "Suicide Rate of Men with AIDS," *Journal of the American Medical Association* 259 (1988):1333–1337; and Kenneth W. Kizer, Martin Green, Carin I. Perkins, Gwendolyn Doebbert, and Michael J. Hughes, "AIDS and Suicide in California," *Journal of the American Medical Association* 260 (1988):1881. These estimates are based on death certificates. Because both suicides and AIDS are underreported on death certificates, these estimates are very conservative.

15. Goffman, *Stigma: Notes on the Management of Spoiled Identity* (Englewood-Cliffs, N.J.: Prentice-Hall, 1963), pp. 41–42.

16. For a discussion of self-blame among other oppressed groups, see Barry Adam, *The Survival of Domination: Inferiorization and Everyday Life* (New York: Elsevier, 1978). For similar findings with regard to persons with HIV disease, see Moulton, "Adjustment to a Diagnosis of AIDS."

17. For a discussion of downward social comparison, see Frederick X. Gibbons, "Stigma and Interpersonal Relationships," in Stephen C. Ainlay, Gaylene Becker, and Lerita M. Coleman, eds., *The Dilemma of Difference: A Multidisciplinary View of Stigma* (New York: Plenum Press, 1986), pp. 123–144.

18. My thanks to Dr. James Allender for these statistics and for helping me understand the neurological implications of HIV disease.

Chapter 5. HIV Disease and the Body

1. R. Nathan Link, Anat R. Feingold, Mitchell H. Charap, Katherine Freeman, and Steven P. Shelov, "Concerns of Medical and Pediatric House Officers about Acquiring AIDS from Their Patients," *American Journal of Public Health* 78 (1988):455–459.

2. Kathryn A. Atchison, Theresa A. Dolan, and Harriette K. Meetz, "Have Dentists Assimilated Information About AIDS?," *Journal of Dental Education* 51 (1987):668–672; Irwin Katz, R. Glen Hass, Nina Parisi, Janetta Astone, and Denise McEvaddy, "Lay People's and Health Care Personnel's Perceptions of Cancer, AIDS, Cardiac, and Diabetic Patients," *Psychological Reports* 60 (1987):615–629; Jeffrey A. Kelly, Janet S. St. Lawrence, Steve Smith, Harold V. Hood, and Donna J. Cook, "Stigmatization of AIDS Patients by Physicians," *American Journal of Public Health* 77 (1987):789–791; and Jean L. Richardson, Thomas Lochner, Kimberly McGuignan, and Alexandra M. Levine, "Physician Attitudes and Experience Regarding the Care of Patients with Acquired Immunodeficiency Syndrome (AIDS) and Related Disorders (ARC)," *Medical Care* 25 (1987):675–685.

3. Barbara Gerbert, Bryan T. Maguire, Stephen B. Hulley, and Thomas J. Coates, "Physicians and Acquired Immunodeficiency Syndrome," *Journal of the American Medical Association* 262 (1989):1969–1972.

4. These costs will be halved if doctors accept the Food and Drug Administration's recent advice to decrease dosages.

5. Peter Aleshire, "AIDS Alters New-Drug Rules," *Arizona Republic,* 27 October 1989.

6. Victor F. Zonana, "AIDS Drug Test Shows 'Serious Promise, Risk,' " Los Angeles *Times,* 20 September 1989, p.A4 + .

7. Erving Goffman, *Presentation of Self in Everyday Life* (Garden City, N.Y.: Doubleday Anchor, 1959), p. 22.

8. For similar findings with regard to other illnesses, see Kathy Charmaz, "Loss of Self: A Fundamental Form of Suffering in the Chronically Ill," *Sociology of Health and Illness* 5 (1983):168–195.

9. For San Francisco data, see Leon McKusick, James Wiley, Thomas Coates, Ronald Stall, Glen Saika, Stephen Morin, Kenneth Charles, William Horstman, and Marcus Conant, "Reported Changes in the Sexual Behavior of Men at Risk for AIDS, San Francisco, 1982–84—The AIDS Behavior Research Project," *Public Health Reports* 100 (1985):622–628. For Arizona data, see Rose Weitz, Shapard Wolf, and Frederick Whitam, "Sexual Knowledge, Attitudes, and Behaviors: A Study of Gay and Bisexual Men in Maricopa County" (Report prepared for Arizona Department of Health Services, 1990).

10. Cheri Register, *Living with Chronic Illness: Days of Patience and Passion* (New York: Free Press, 1987).

11. Personal communication, Dr. James Allender.

12. Personal communication, Dr. James Allender.

13. For similar findings with regard to other illness, see Nancy A. Brooks and Ronald R. Matson, "Managing Multiple Sclerosis," *Research in the Sociology of Health Care* 6 (1987):73–106.

14. For similar findings with regard to other illnesses, see Brooks and Matson, "Managing Multiple Sclerosis"; Bury, "Chronic Illness as Biographical Disruption"; Charmaz, *The Social Reality of Death* (Reading, Mass.: Addison-Wesley, 1980), pp. 155–170; Charmaz, "Loss of Self"; Charmaz, "Struggling for a Self: Identity Levels of the Chronically Ill," *Research in the Sociology of Health Care* 6 (1987):283–321; Juliet Corbin and Anselm L. Strauss, "Accompaniments of Chronic Illness: Changes in Body, Self, Biography, and Biographical Time," *Research in the Sociology of Health Care* 6 (1987):249–282; and Joseph Schneider and Peter Conrad, *Having Epilepsy: The Experience and Control of Illness,* (Philadelphia: Temple University Press, 1983).

15. Compare to Peter Conrad, "The Meaning of Medications: Another Look at Compliance," *Social Science and Medicine* 20 (1985):29–37; Goffman, *Stigma: Notes on the Management of Spoiled Identity* (Englewood Cliffs, N.J.: Prentice-Hall, 1963); Nancy G. Kutner, "Social Worlds and Identity in End-stage Renal Disease (ESRD)," *Research in the Sociology of Health Care* 6 (1987):33–71; and Mark Peyrot, James F. McMurry, Jr., and Richard Hedges, "Living with Diabetes: The Role of Personal and Professional Knowledge in Symptom and Regimen Management," *Research in the Sociology of Health Care* 6 (1987):107–146.

16. Charmaz, *The Social Reality of Death* and Charmaz, "Loss of Self."

Chapter 6. HIV Disease and Social Relationships

1. Arthur S. Leonard, "AIDS in the Workplace," in Harlon L. Dalton, Scott Burris, and the Yale AIDS Law Project, eds., *AIDS and the Law: A Guide for the Public* (New Haven: Yale University Press, 1987), pp. 109–125.

Chapter 7. Making a Life with HIV Disease

1. See, for example: Marie I. Boutte, " 'The Stumbling Disease': A Case Study of Stigma Among Azorean-Portuguese," *Social Science and Medicine* 24 (1987):209–217; Richard A. Hilbert, "The Acultural Dimensions of Chronic Pain: Flawed Reality Construction and the Problem of Meaning," *Social Problems* 31 (1984):365–378; and Joseph Schneider and Peter Conrad, *Having Epilepsy: The Experience and Control of Illness* (Philadelphia: Temple University Press, 1983).

2. See, for example: Zachary Gussow and George S. Tracy, "Status, Ideology, and Adaptation to Stigmatized Illness: A Study of Leprosy," *Human Organization* 27 (1968):316–325; and John Kitsuse, "Coming Out All Over: Deviants and the Politics of Social Problems," *Social Problems* 28 (1980):1–13.

3. Erving Goffman, *Relations in Public* (New York: Basic Books, 1971).

4. This research is summarized in Viktor Gecas, "The Self-Concept," *Annual Review of Sociology* 8 (1982):1–33; and Barry R. Schlenker, *The Self and Social Life* (New York: McGraw-Hill, 1985), pp. 12–15, 89–92.

5. See Appendix 1 for further details.

6. My thanks to Kathy Charmaz for helping me conceptualize this section.

7. Kathy Charmaz, "Struggling for a Self: Identity Levels of the Chronically Ill," *Research in the Sociology of Health Care* 6 (1987):283–321.

8. Gussow and Tracy, "Status, Ideology, and Adaptation to Stigmatized Illness."

9. Charmaz, "Struggling for a Self."

Chapter 8. The Doctors' Perspectives

1. See George J. Annas, "Legal Risks and Responsibilities of Physicians in the AIDS Epidemic," *Hastings Center Report* 18 (1988):26–32; Taunya L. Banks, "The Right to Medical Treatment," in Harlon L. Dalton, Scott Burris, and the Yale AIDS Project, eds., *AIDS and the Law* (New Haven: Yale University Press, 1987), pp. 175–184; and Mary K.

Logan, "Legal, Ethical Issues for Dentists," *Journal of the American Dental Association* 115 (1987):402.

2. American Dental Association, *Policy Statement on AIDS, HIV Infection and the Practice of Dentistry* (Chicago, 1988); and Council on Ethical and Judicial Affairs, "Ethical Issues Involved in the Growing AIDS Crisis," *Journal of the American Medical Association* 259 (1988):1360–1361.

3. Annas, "Legal Risks and Responsibilities," p. 30; American Dental Association, personal communication, 1988.

4. Kathryn A. Atchison, Theresa A. Dolan, and Harriette K. Meetz, "Have Dentists Assimilated Information About AIDS?," *Journal of Dental Education* 51 (1987):668–672.

5. Jean L. Richardson, Thomas Lochner, Kimberly McGuignan, and Alexandra M. Levine, "Physician Attitudes and Experience Regarding the Care of Patients with Acquired Immunodeficiency Syndrome (AIDS) and Related Disorders (ARC)," *Medical Care* 25 (1987):675–685.

6. For similar conclusions, see Helen E. Dosik, "The AIDS Doctors: Caught in the Uncertainties of a Contaminating Disease" (Paper presented at the American Sociological Association meetings, 1987).

7. R. Nathan Link, Anat R. Feingold, Mitchell H. Charap, Katherine Freeman, and Steven P. Shelov, "Concerns of Medical and Pediatric House Officers About Acquiring AIDS from Their Patients," *American Journal of Public Health* 78 (1988):455–459.

8. Some of these reasons are discussed briefly in Leon McKusick, William Horstman, Donald Abrams, and Thomas J. Coates, "Psychological Impact of AIDS on Primary Care Physicians," *Western Journal of Medicine* 144 (1986):751–752.

9. Link et al., "Concerns of Medical and Pediatric House Officers."

10. McKusick et al., "Psychological Impact of AIDS on Primary Care Physicians."

11. Richard Belitsky and Robert A. Solomon, "Doctors and Patients: Responsibilities in a Confidential Relationship," in Dalton, Burris, and the Yale AIDS Project, eds., *AIDS and the Law*, pp. 201–209; Council on Ethical and Judicial Affairs, "Ethical Issues Involved in the Growing AIDS Crisis"; and Helen M. Cole, "Legal Limits of AIDS Confidentiality," *Journal of the American Medical Association* 259 (1988):3449–3451.

12. For similar findings, see Dosik, "The AIDS Doctors"; and Robert M. Wachter, "The Impact of the Acquired Immunodeficiency Syn-

drome on Medical Residency Training," *New England Journal of Medicine* 314 (1986):177–180.

13. McKusick et al., "Psychological Impact of AIDS on Primary Care Physicians."

14. Robert Steinbrook, Bernard Lo, Jill Tirpack, James Dilley, and Paul Volberding, "Ethical Dilemmas in Caring for Patients with the Acquired Immunodeficiency Syndrome," *Annals of Internal Medicine* 103 (1985):787–790.

15. For further discussion of this issue see Molly Cooke, "Ethical Issues in the Care of Patients with AIDS," *Quality Review Bulletin* 12 (1986):343–346; and Bernard Lo, Thomas A. Raffin, Neal H. Cohen, Robert M. Wachter, John M. Luce, and Philip C. Hopewell, "Ethical Dilemmas about Intensive Care for Patients with AIDS," *Reviews of Infectious Diseases* 9 (1987):1163–1167.

16. For further discussion, see Steinbrook et al., "Ethical Dilemmas in Caring for Patients."

Chapter 9. The Future of HIV

1. This discussion draws heavily on Thomas J. Matthews and Dani P. Bolognesi, "AIDS Vaccines," *Scientific American* 259, no. 40 (1988):110–119; and Institute of Medicine, National Academy of Sciences, *Confronting AIDS: Update 1988* (Washington, D.C.: National Academy Press, 1988).

2. Figures taken from "AIDS and Human Immunodeficiency Virus Infection in the United States: 1988 Update," *Morbidity and Mortality Weekly Report* 38 (supplement), 12 May 1989. The federal government only keeps records of persons with AIDS, not all persons with HIV disease.

3. Centers for Disease Control, *HIV/AIDS Surveillance Report* (Atlanta, Ga.: Centers for Disease Control, December 1989) and Centers for Disease Control, *AIDS Weekly Surveillance Report* (Atlanta, Ga.: Centers for Disease Control, 1 December 1986).

4. Gerald Friedland, "Parenteral Drug Users," in Richard A. Kaslow and Donald P. Francis, eds., *The Epidemiology of AIDS: Expression, Occurrence, and Control of Human Immunodeficiency Virus Type 1 Infection* (New York: Oxford University Press, 1989), pp. 153–178.

5. Institute of Medicine, *Confronting AIDS,* p. 52.

6. For persons with HIV disease, see *Morbidity and Mortality Weekly Report,* 1989, p. 2. For the U.S. population, see U.S. Bureau of the Census, *Statistical Abstract of the United States* (Washington, D.C.: Government Printing Office, 1989), p. 131.

7. Institute of Medicine, *Confronting AIDS,* p. 40.

8. For discussions of the costs of screening see, for example: Michael J. Barry, Paul D. Cleary, and Harvey V. Fineberg, "Screening for HIV Infection: Risks, Benefits, and the Burden of Proof," *Law, Medicine and Health Care* 14 (1986):259–267; Paul D. Cleary, Michael J. Barry, Kenneth H. Mayer, Allan M. Brandt, Larry Gostin, and Harvey V. Fineberg, "Compulsory Premarital Screening for the Human Immunodeficiency Virus: Technical and Public Health Considerations," *Journal of the American Medical Association* 258 (1987):1757–1762; Klemens B. Meyer and Stephen G. Pauker, "Screening for HIV: Can We Afford the False Positive Rate?" *New England Journal of Medicine* 317 (1987):238–241; and Bernard J. Turnock and Chester J. Kelly, "Mandatory Premarital Testing for Human Immunodeficiency Virus: The Illinois Experience," *Journal of the American Medical Association* 261 (1989):3415–3418.

9. See, for example, Sandra G. Boodman, "AIDS Tests Often Performed Without Patients' Knowledge," *Washington Post,* 21 November 1988, p.A1 + ; and Keith Henry, Karen Willenbring, and Kent Crossley, "Human Immunodeficiency Virus Antibody Testing," *Journal of The American Medical Association* 259 (1988):1819–1822.

10. Peter S. Arno, Douglas Shenson, Naomi F. Siegel, Pat Franks, and Philip R. Lee, "Economic and Policy Implications of Early Intervention in HIV Disease," *Journal of the American Medical Association* 262 (1989):1493–1498.

11. Ibid.

12. Larry Gostin and Andrew Ziegler, "A Review of AIDS-Related Legislative and Regulatory Policy in the United States," *Law, Medicine, and Health Care* 15 (1987):5–16.

13. Charles L. Bennett, Jeffrey B. Garfinkle, Sheldon Greenfield, David Draper, William Rogers, W. Christopher Matthews, and David E. Kanouse, "The Relation Between Hospital Experience and In-Hospital Mortality for Patients with AIDS-Related PCP," *Journal of the American Medical Association* 261 (1989):2975–2979. However, Deborah J. Cotton, "Improving Survival in Acquired Immunodeficiency Syndrome: Is Experi-

ence Everything?" *Journal of the American Medical Association* 261 (1989):3016–3017, suggests that more data are needed before we can generalize from Bennett's findings.

14. Gloria Kapantais and Eve Powell-Griner, "Characteristics of Persons Dying from AIDS: Preliminary Data from the 1986 National Mortality Followback Survey," *Advance Data from Vital and Health Statistics* No. 173 (Hyattsville, Md.: National Center for Health Statistics, 1989).

15. Harvey V. Fineberg, "The Social Dimensions of AIDS," *Scientific American* 259 (October 1988), 128–134.

16. See David E. Bloom and Geoffrey Carliner, "The Economic Impact of AIDS in the United States," *Science* 239 (1988):604–610; Benjamin Schatz, *HIV Testing by Insurers: Profits Versus the Public Good* (Testimony submitted to the U.S. Commission on Civil Rights, 27 April 1988); and Mark Scherzer, "Insurance," in Harlon L. Dalton, Scott Burris, and the Yale AIDS Law Project, eds., *AIDS and the Law: A Guide for the Public* (New Haven: Yale University Press, 1987), pp. 185–200.

17. Peter S. Arno, "The Economic Impact of AIDS," *Journal of the American Medical Association* 258 (1987):1376–1377.

18. Ibid., p. 1377.

19. Figures on the costs of treating HIV disease taken from Dennis P. Andrulis, Virginia Beers Weslowski, and Larry S. Gage, "The 1987 US Hospital AIDS Survey," *Journal of the American Medical Association* 262 (1989):784–794.

20. Institute of Medicine, *Confronting AIDS,* pp. 104–106.

21. U.S. Bureau of the Census, *Statistical Abstract,* p. 449.

22. Centers for Disease Control, *HIV/AIDS Surveillance Report* (1989), p. 6.

23. For further details, see Ann A. Scitovsky, Mary Cline, and Philip R. Lee, "Medical Care Costs of Patients with AIDS in San Francisco," *Journal of the American Medical Association* 256 (1986):3103–3106; and Arno, "The Nonprofit Sector's Response to the AIDS Epidemic: Community-based Services in San Francisco," *American Journal of Public Health* 76 (1986):1325–1330.

24. See Arno, "The Nonprofit Sector's Response."

25. Personal communication, Eric Engstrom, Executive Director, National AIDS Network, April 1990.

26. For further discussion, see Deborah J. Cotton, "The Impact of

AIDS on the Medical Care System," *Journal of the American Medical Association* 260 (1988):519–523.

27. Molly Cooke and Merle A. Sande, "The HIV Epidemic and Training in Internal Medicine: Challenges and Recommendations," *New England Journal of Medicine* 321 (1989):1334–1338.

28. For example, see David Sudnow, *Passing On: The Social Organization of Dying* (Englewood Cliffs, N.J.: Prentice-Hall, 1967).

29. National Institute for Occupational Safety and Health, *Guidelines for Preventing the Transmission of HIV and HBV to Health Care and Public Safety Workers* (Atlanta, Ga.: Centers for Disease Control, 1989), p. 24.

30. This discussion draws heavily on Robert Yarchoan, Hiroaki Mitsuya, and Samuel Broder, "AIDS Therapies," *Scientific American* 259, no. 40 (1988):110–119.

31. Michael Specter, "1989 was Year of Gains for AIDS Research," *Arizona Republic*, 1 January 1990, p. A4.

32. Division of AIDS, *Results of Controlled Clinical Trials of Zidovudine in Early HIV Infection* (Bethesda, Md.: National Institute of Allergy and Infectious Diseases, 29 August 1989).

Appendix 1

1. I subsequently learned, however, that sociologists' rights are greater in circumstances such as my own where the researcher consistently has emphasized to subjects that the data will be kept confidential and has established procedures to ensure this. See Ronald Bayer, Carol Levine, and Thomas H. Murray, "Guidelines for Confidentiality in Research on AIDS," *IRB: A Review of Human Subjects Research* 6 (1984):1–7.

Appendix 2

1. Arizona Department of Health Services, *Definitive and Presumptive AIDS cases in Arizona and AIDS Related Complex (ARC): Surveillance Report for Arizona* (December 1989).

Index

Report (continued)
Virus Epidemic (Office of Technology Assessment), 29
research, 5, 33, 74; funding for, 28–29; sociological, 187–194; into treatment, 182–183; on vaccines, 165–167
retroviruses, 165–166, 181
risk groups, 53, 168–169; definition of, 13–14; perception of, 14–15
Rueda, Enrique, 22

San Francisco, 10, 53, 88, 173; public health care in, 176–178
School Board of Nassau County v. *Arline,* 31–32
Schwartz, Michael, 22
secrecy, about illness, 104, 106–107, 117, 128–130, 145. *See also* shame; stigma
segregation, 27
self-concept, 135; changes in, 91–94, 99–101, 137, 145–146
self-esteem, 96–97, 137; improving, 139–140; maintaining, 135–136, 138
sexual behavior, 5, 12, 15, 69–70; safer, 30–31
sexuality, 70; changes in, 92–94, 136; of gay men, 139–140; and stigmatized illness, 46–47
shame, 96, 104, 135. *See also* secrecy; stigma
Siegel, Bernie, *Love, Medicine and Miracles,* 43
social services, provision of, 158–160

spouses, relationships with, 109–116
standard of living, 96
stigma, 172, 181; avoidance of, 128–132, 145; disclosure and, 129–130; of family, 105–106; illness as, 34, 43–44, 45–48, 126–127; reduction of, 132–134; in workplace, 123–124, 125–126. *See also* secrecy; shame
stress, 54, 94, 102, 141, 161
subcultures, 5
suicide, 66
support groups, 173; participation in, 74, 75, 77, 130–132. *See also* counseling
survey, confidentiality of, 191–194
symptoms, 8, 129; of HIV disease, 60–63

testing, 170, 172, 174; for HIV, 56–59, 170; recommending, 151–153; reporting results of, 153–154, 188
transfusions, 15–16, 53, 62
transmission: awareness of, 53–55; of HIV, 15–16, 18, 19–20, 52, 168–170, 200–201n11. *See also* contagion; infection
treatment, 85, 181; alternative, 49–51, 89; attitude toward, 88–89; after diagnosis, 64–67; and doctors' attitudes, 147–149; drug therapy as, 86–88, 156–158; of dying patients, 160–162; prospects for, 181–